Homemade Beauty Products for Beginners

The Complete Bundle Guide to Making Luxurious Homemade Body Butter, Homemade Soap, Homemade Shampoo & Homemade Bath Bombs

Introduction

Beauty products are something every girl needs in today's world. The problem is, it would burn a hole in our pockets if we were to buy EVERY single beauty product we need and want from today's leading beauty stores. Plus, most of them are filled with chemicals that are actually very dangerous to our skin and overall health.

From body butters to soaps to shampoos, I'm here to tell you that there ARE ways to still look beautiful and take care of yourself, without throwing your money down the drain or sacrificing your health for beauty.

The solution? Homemade beauty products! The simple answer is, you can make most of the products you need yourself, right at home. All you need is a little know-how and a little time. Most of the ingredients needed probably already exist somewhere in your pantry – and if not, they're pretty cheap to buy compared to the money you'd be spending on fancy commercialized products.

This book comes to you from best-selling Kindle author Karen Wells, and is a bundle compilation of 4 books Karen has written:

1. Homemade Body Butter: Over 25 Rejuvenating Body Butter & Body Scrub Recipes to Give You Soft, Glowing Skin
2. Soap Making: Homemade Soap for Beginners - The Complete Guide to Making Luxurious, Skin-Softening Soap at Home
3. Homemade Shampoo: Over 25 Revitalizing, Natural Shampoo Recipes to Give You Healthy, Beautiful Hair
4. Homemade Bath Bombs: The Complete DIY Guide to Making Luxurious, Soothing Bath Bombs

This book offers you the opportunity to read ALL 4 books so that you get a complete guide on making homemade beauty products from start to finish. Read on, and enjoy!

Table of Contents:

Book 1:
Homemade Body Butters

Over 25 Rejuvenating Body Butter &
Body Scrub Recipes to Give You Soft,
Glowing Skin

Karen Wells

Introduction

Welcome! I want to thank you again for downloading this book, and I'm glad you're interested in learning how to make homemade body butter and homemade body scrubs for yourself – your body will love you for it!

Homemade body scrubs and body butters can have a magical effect on your body, mind, and spirit. The health benefits of applying ingredients on your skin such as olive oil, coconut oil, honey and lemon are staggering (and maybe even shocking)...I can't wait for you to learn about them in this book!

When using homemade body butter recipes and homemade body scrubs, not only are you beautifying your skin; but you are also absorbing antioxidants, enhancing your skin's UV resistance, and stimulating your immune system just to name a few benefits. These natural ingredients (most of which you already have in your kitchen) will make you love your skin and your body even more!

Isn't that the bigger picture here? By treating your body right – easing irritable skin, soothing your mind with lavender oil or honey, and revitalizing the dead surfaces of your skin – you are embracing your true beauty and nurturing your body. Nothing is more beautiful than that!

As you may have guessed, this book is for beginners who want to learn how to make their skin naturally glow with radiance, using gentle and healthy homemade products. So as you read this book and start to make your own natural body butters, scrubs and masks, my hope is that your inner beauty will shine through as you become healthier and more confident with your skin!

Table of Contents

The Wondrous Benefits of Homemade Body Butters & Scrubs

Have you ever felt like you just can't get rid of dry, dull skin? For many of us it's a constant problem. Of course, that's not what we want for ourselves! We want glowing, beautiful skin 24/7 – but it seems that dry winter weather, harsh chemical-laden soaps, and a slew of other factors would like to tell us otherwise. The worst part is that many of the so-called "moisturizing" soaps, lotions, and scrubs that you buy at the store actually do you more harm than good. We'll get more into that in the next section, but for now we can agree that it's definitely a struggle to take better care of our skin and something needs to be done about it! So now, let's take a look at how natural homemade body butters and scrubs address this problem and how they can nourish, hydrate, and beautify our skin!

Simply put, the ingredients that make up homemade, natural body butters and scrubs work hard to make you beautiful. Their moisturizing and hydrating properties protect your skin and leave it soft and pure. The most common ingredients used such as coconut oil, olive oil, shea butter, lemon, lavender and oatmeal contain antibacterial, antiviral, and anti-fungal properties. They are antioxidants too, which means that while making the surface of your skin clear and vibrant, they are working on your cells too! They help to fight free radicals and protect you from infections.

Natural homemade scrubs and lotions also help clear skin irritations and leave your skin feeling and looking youthful! Honey encourages wound healing and can reduce breakouts, rosemary is a good source of iron and calcium, and vanilla is an aphrodisiac, as it has a pleasing affect on your mind and body. These simple household ingredients will leave you with beautiful and healthy skin – isn't it amazing to see how helpful natural ingredients can be? You will learn to love trying new ingredients and discovering their magic by the time you're done reading this book!

Additionally, salt and sugar scrubs are one of easiest home treatments that truly deliver. Not only is slathering sugar and oil all over your body a moment of personal love and devotion, but the exfoliating factor leaves your skin refreshed, vibrant, and smooth.

Lastly, let's also look at the impact homemade beauty products can have on your self-esteem. By mixing up your own remedy, rubbing it onto your skin, and watching the beautiful and sometimes jaw-dropping outcome of these ingredients, you are really experiencing a moment of self-love. I want you to love yourself and your body enough to treat it to a delicious Soft-Served Vanilla Body Butter or a Banana Foster Body Scrub. You are having a moment with yourself! When you see the skin-deep effects of these moisturizing and relaxing ingredients you'll boost your confidence, and there's nothing more important than that.

Why Homemade Body Butters & Scrubs Instead of Store-Bought?

The best thing about making your own, homemade body scrub or lotion is that you control what goes into it! You decide on every component of your product, and you get to choose your favorite ingredients. Many homemade scrubs only need a few ingredients, and they are easy to find. Citrus fruits, bananas, lemons, or household herbs – you pick what you love most and add it in!

Further, these homemade concoctions can be more affordable – they are actually downright cheap. With just a few dollars you can choose your own ingredients and be aware of what exactly is being used on your skin.

Here are a few noteworthy and unnerving facts on store-bought beauty products... To start, the regulation of cosmetic and personal-care products is slim – the process is very easy to get approved. Because of this, the ingredient labels can be downright scary! There are probably thousands of chemicals throughout the products you own – and every time you use them, they are being absorbed into your body. There is little government review or approvals involved because the industry is highly unregulated.

The majority of commercial skin care and beauty products, including scrubs, use inorganic compounds and petroleum-based gels as their foundation. Mineral oils are not naturally harvested from plants. When an ingredient is made with chemicals, it actually clogs your pores. Your skin loses its natural ability to expel toxins, which actually leads to increased acne and signs of aging! Putting chemicals on your body will limit your skin's natural healing processes. Even further – your body's immune system, the health of your eyes, and your respiratory system can be damaged by unhealthy chemicals and additives in your products. Also, many of these chemicals are skin irritants.

It's sad, but commercial scrubs and lotions typically contain toxic ingredients and chemical fragrances that are linked to all sorts of issues, from allergies to cancer. A few harmful chemicals that are used in store-bought washes, scrubs and lotions include parabens (used for preservation), synthetic colors (derived from petroleum or coal tar sources), artificial fragrance (which is associated with allergies and respiratory distress), toluene (which is also used to dissolve paint), and sodium lauryl sulfate or SLS (which can cause kidney and respiratory damage). These are just a few of the chemicals that are used! If the goal of using these products is to look and feel beautiful, then this could be a problem.

Last, it is also better for the environment to make your own scrubs and lotions. Petroleum-based oils are made from unsustainable fossil fuel. Also, the plastic packaging is a huge waste – think of all those plastic jars and bottles!

You use skin scrubs and body butters to make your skin look and feel beautiful. You love the smell and the texture of these products. Then why not take full advantage of the benefits of making these products on your own? They're healthier, and can be less expensive, and you know exactly what's going onto your skin!

The Basics for Beginners: What You Need to Know to Get Started

By now, you probably have decided to create your very own body butters or scrubs because you want to treat your body right! After applying the recipes in this book, it won't take long for you to notice that your skin is smoother, looks brighter, glows more, and has less irritations or signs of acne. Once you begin playing with ingredients to make your own unique mixture for your skin type, you will never go back! Here are a few more tips, pointers, and things you should know before we dive into the recipes.

The Cleansing Properties of Oil:

Cleaning your face and body with oil may seem strange, since so many people associate oil with greasy and dirty skin, but the truth is that oil cleansing is a great way to wash your body. It naturally cleanses and dissolves the bad oils on your skin, without drying out the delicate facial skin area. Many scrub and butter recipes call for olive oil, coconut oil, almond oil, and essential oils. Try to find organic brands when purchasing these oils because there will be virtually no additives. Also, when choosing essential oils, think about what mood or feeling you are trying to achieve when using your product. For example, if you are looking for a soothing and calming fragrance, then go with lavender. If you want to be invigorated by your scrub or butter, then choose lemon or rosemary. So don't be afraid to use oils!

Benefits of Exfoliating Your Skin with Scrubs:

Exfoliating your skin will keep it healthy because it helps get rid of dead skin and it draws out other impurities and bacterias. Some natural exfoliating ingredients include coarse salt and sugar, coffee grounds, and oatmeal. This will invigorate your skin and keep it looking and feeling fresh.

Hydrating Your Skin with Body Butters:

Hydrating your skin helps you to protect the surface of your body from the outside world, as it seals in the beneficial effects of these natural ingredients and it keeps your skin smooth. Banana, honey, and avocado are natural ingredients that contain vitamins and hydrating properties.

Using Face Masks:

Face masks help treat particular skin types and conditions. Homemade face masks are easy to make, regardless of your skin type – whether it's dry (use an ingredient like avocado), irritated (use lemon or honey), or oily (use apple cider vinegar). Who would've known? There are so many naturally healing ingredients in your kitchen, and you didn't even know it!

Storing Your Recipes:

For storage, you can simply store your scrubs and body butters in glass jars with a lid! Wide-mouth mason jars work great for this. Once you've created your recipe, store it in a cool, dark place (no direct sunlight). Specific instructions for storage will be given with each recipe later. Also, try to use your recipes within 1-2 weeks from creating them.

Tools/Equipment Needed:

When making body butters, many recipes call for a blender or an attachable whisk. Use whatever you have at home – even if you need to hand-whip your lotions. It may take a little longer, but it will work! If you need to grind an ingredient, you can use a blender, a food processor, or a coffee grinder – again, whatever you have at home will do just fine. The recipes in this book are fairly easy to get started and don't require any fancy equipment other than standard household items like those listed here.

Most of all, enjoy playing with these beautifying mixtures and have fun!

Body Butter Recipes

Whipped Coconut-Creme Oil

This body butter oil mixture will have you smelling like an island breeze in no time. Its fluffy texture is perfect for moisturizing your body from head to toe.

Estimated time: 10 minutes

1 cup of coconut oil

2 tablespoons of jojoba oil

1 teaspoon of vitamin E oil

10-15 drops of vanilla essential oil

1. Oh high speed, whip together coconut oil, jojoba oil and vitamin E oil for about 8 minutes, until light and fluffy.

2. Wipe the sides every minute or so to get everything really mixed together.

3. Add the vanilla essential oil at the end and then whip the mixture for another 30 seconds.

4. Store in a clean jar with a lid. Does not need to be refrigerated.

Tropical Body Butter

This sweet and tropical body butter will tempt you to change into your bikini. It smells like paradise and it contains antioxidants.

Estimated time: 90 minutes (including waiting time)

1/2 cup Shea Butter

1/2 cup of Mango Butter

1/2 cup of Coconut Oil

1/2 cup of almond oil

15 drops of citrus essential oil

1. In a glass bowl, combine all ingredients except for the citrus essential oil.

2. Bring the mixture to medium heat and stir it constantly until all ingredients are melted.

3. Remove the mixture from the heat and let it cool slightly.

4. Move the mixture to the refrigerator and let it cool for about an hour, or until it begins to harden.

5. Add the citrus oil and then use a hand mixer to whip the mixture for 10 minutes, or until fluffy.

6. Return the mixture to the refrigerator for 10-15 minutes.

7. Store your body butter in a glass jar with a lid and keep it in a cool place.

Soft-Serve Vanilla Body Butter

Treat yourself to this moisturizing and skin-enriching body butter that smells like dessert.

Estimated time: 90 minutes (including waiting time)

1 cup raw Cocoa Butter

1/2 cup of sweet almond oil

1/2 cup of Coconut Oil

1 vanilla bean

1. Melt cocoa butter and coconut oil, then remove the mixture from heat and let it cool for 30 minutes.

2. Grind a vanilla bean in a coffee grinder, or a food processor.

3. Stir sweet almond oil and vanilla bean bits into the cocoa butter and coconut oil mixture.

4. Place the mixture in the freezer to chill for about 20 minutes.

5. Whip with an electric mixer, or a food processor, until the mixture becomes a buttery consistency.

6. Store your body butter in a jar with a lid and keep it in a cool place.

Sweet Peppermint Body Butter

This fresh and sweet body butter will invigorate your skin and it serves as an antibacterial agent.

Estimated time: 70 minutes (including waiting time)

1/2 cup Coconut Oil

1/2 cup Cocoa Butter

1/2 cup Shea Butter

1/2 cup sweet almond oil

1 teaspoon of vitamin E oil

2-4 drops of peppermint essential oil

1. Place coconut oil, cocoa butter, and shea butter in a medium sized pot over low heat. Stir to combine until it melts completely, then remove the mixture from heat.

2. Thoroughly mix in the sweet almond oil, vitamin E oil, and peppermint oil.

3. Chill the mixture in your refrigerator for an hour, until it becomes firm, but not hard.

4. Use a mixer until you have created a whipped consistency.

5. Store your body butter in a jar with a lid and keep it in a cool place.

Lemon Drop Body Butter

This body butter is perfect for dry skin; it will leave your skin feeling soft and hydrated.

Estimated time: 70 minutes (including waiting time)

6 tablespoons of Coconut Oil

1 tablespoon of Vitamin E oil

1/4 teaspoon of lemon essential oil

1/4 cup of Cocoa Butter

1. Heat the coconut oil and cocoa butter until the mixture comes together.

2. Place the mixture in the freezer for about an hour, until it becomes firm, but not hard.

3. Add in the Vitamin E oil and lemon essential oil.

4. Use a mixer until you have created a whipped consistency.

5. Store your body butter in a jar with a lid and keep it in a cool place.

Rosemary Mint Body Butter

This lotion made of Shea Butter helps to heal burns, scars and sores – it can even diminish wrinkles!

Estimated time: 60 minutes

3 tablespoons of Cocoa Butter

6 tablespoons of Shea Butter

3 tablespoons of Kukui Nut Oil

20 drops of spearmint essential oil

10 drops of rosemary essential oil

1. In a medium sized glass bowl, add in the Cocoa Butter, Shea Butter, and Kukui Nut Oil. Place the bowl over a pan of simmering water and allow the butters to melt together.

2. Let the mixture cool at room temperature for 10 minutes, then put it in the freezer for 20 minutes.

3. Blend the mixture with a whisk attachment for 5 minutes, then put it back in the freezer.

4. Repeat step 3 until the mixture turns into a creamy color.

5. Store your body butter in a jar with a lid and keep it in a cool place.

Coconut Lavender Body Butter

The scent of lavender is soothing and relaxing, and the Coconut Oil will strengthen your underlying tissue. This body butter will leave you feeling beautiful from within!

Estimated time: 30 minutes

4 tablespoons of Coconut Oil

1 tablespoon of Jojoba Oil

1/2 tablespoon of lavender infused oil

10 drops of rose essential oil

1. Place the Coconut Oil, Jojoba Oil, and lavender infused oil in a glass bowl.

2. Heat the mixture over a pan of simmering water until the coconut oil is melted.

3. Whisk the ingredients together, then allow the mixture to cool to room temperature.

4. Once the mixture is cooled, add in the rose oil and whisk until fluffy.

Infused Rosemary and Orange Body Butter

This natural and soothing body butter will allow your skin to absorb all of its moisturizing and hydrating properties.

Estimated time: 90 minutes (including waiting time)

1 cup of Shea Butter

1/2 cup of Coconut oil

1/2 cup almond oil

Pinch of fresh rosemary

Peel from one orange

1. Infuse the rosemary and orange peel by letting it steep in hot water for 30 minutes.

2. In the meantime, melt the Shea Butter and Coconut Oil. Let it cool for 30 minutes, then stir in the almond oil.

3. Use a stainer to drain the rosemary and orange peel. Add about 2 teaspoons of infused water to the mixture.

4. Let the mixture chill outside or in the freezer, wait until the oil begins to solidify.

5. Whip the mixture until you have achieved a buttery consistency.

6. Place in a jar with a lid and keep your body butter in a cool place.

Coconut and Beeswax Lotion Bars

These lotion bars are a nice alternative to jarred lotion. You rub it on your skin and your body heat will melt the oils, absorbing these hydrating qualities into the skin.

Estimated time: 60 minutes (including waiting time)

1/4 cup Beeswax, grated

1/4 cup Cocoa Butter, grated

1/3 cup Coconut Oil

1 tablespoon Almond Oil

1 tablespoon Jojoba Oil

1. In a microwave-safe bowl, heat the beeswax and cocoa butter in short bursts (30 seconds each) until they melt.

2. Whisk the mixture together and then add the oils.

3. Pour the mixture into muffin tins lined with paper baking cups.

4. Place in the refrigerator (or freezer) until set.

Rose Oil Infused Coco Butter

Allow yourself to indulge in this aromatic body butter. Feel good and smell good like Cleopatra after using this recipe!

Estimated time: 50 minutes (including waiting time)

¼ cup refined coconut oil

10 drops rose essential oil

½ tbsp. Jojoba oil

3 drops Alkanets infused oil

¼ tbsp. cornstarch

1. In a glass bowl, combine the refined coconut oil, Alkanet, and cornstarch.
2. Place the bowl over simmering water until the coco oil has melted.
3. Whisk all the ingredients together.
4. Allow to cool in room temperature before adding the rose essential oil.
5. Whisk again before storing in an air tight jar.
6. You can use the coco butter up to 3 months.

Honey-Pineapple Body Butter

Be beach ready with this body butter recipe made with pineapple essential oil and honey. This recipe is smells so yummy, you'll be tempted to eat it!

Estimated time: 50 minutes (including waiting time)

15 drops pineapple essential oil

2 tbsp. pure honey

½ cup Shea butter

2 tbsp. beeswax

1/3 cup coconut oil

10 drops coconut essential oil

1/3 cup jojoba oil

1. Combine in a glass bowl the honey, Shea butter, coconut oil, and beeswax.
2. Transfer the mixture on a double boiler, or place the bowl on top of simmering water.
3. Once the mixture has melted, remove the bowl from the heat and then pour the jojoba oil in. Mix well.

4. Add the pineapple essential oil as well as the coconut essential oil.

5. Place the mixture in the fridge to chill for 30 minutes.

6. After 30 mins, whip the mixture before storing in an air-tight container.

3-Ingredient Citrus Body Butter

Everybody loves the scent of citrusy fruits, so you'll definitely fall in love with this simple coco body butter recipe. This recipe uses honey as one of its ingredients which is proven to moisturize the skin and create a healthy glow.

Estimated time: 45 minutes (including waiting time)

2 tbsp. zest of grapefruit

1 ½ cup coconut oil

3 tbsp. pure honey

1. Melt the coconut oil in a glass bowl on top of simmering water. Allow to the coco oil to melt for a 10 minutes while stirring occasionally.

2. Remove the bowl from the heat and then immediately add in the zest and honey. Combine well.

3. Place the mixture in the fridge to cool down for 30 minutes.

4. Once cooled, whisk the mixture using a hand mixer to achieve a butter-like texture.

(This recipe can last for only 1-2 months because of the citrus zest.)

Aromatic Avocado Body Butter

Not only is avocado healthy a fruit for consumption, but its oil can also do wonders for our skin. Avocado is rich in vitamins A, C, and E that promotes healthy skin cells. Enjoy this avocado recipe infused with lavender essential oil.

Estimated time: 30 minutes

1 cup avocado oil

12 drops lavender essential oil

1 cup Shea oil

3 tsp. cornstarch

1. Melt the Shea butter in a glass bowl placed on top of a pot of simmering water while stirring occasionally. (You can also use a double boiler for this.)

2. Remove the mixture from the heat when the Shea butter has melted. Add the lavender oil, avocado oil and then the cornstarch. Combine well.

3. Place the glass bowl in a prepared (larger) bowl with iced water. As the mixture cools, whisk the ingredients together using a hand mixture until you achieve a butter-like texture.

4. Transfer the body butter in a sterilized, air-tight container.

Invigorating Rosehip Body Butter

Bring back your skin's youth with this skin-tightening body butter recipe.

Estimated time: 3.5 hours (including waiting time)

2 tbsp. rosehip oil

2 tbsp. arnica essential oil

½ cup Shea butter

½ cup kokum butter

¼ cup avocado oil

½ cup coconut oil

1. Place all the ingredients in a glass bowl.

2. Combine and melt them by placing the bowl on top of a simmering pot of water; stir occasionally.

3. Remove the bowl from the heat when the ingredients are melted and are well incorporated. Place the bowl in the fridge to chill for 3 hours.

4. After 3 hours, remove the mixture from the fridge and whip using a mixture for 15 minutes or until the texture begins to become like a frosting.

5. Transfer the body butter in a jar and store in a dry room with no direct sunlight.

Stress-busting Body Butter

Indeed. Besides keeping your skin smooth and healthy, this body butter recipe can relieve you from stress because of the magnesium flakes' effect of lowering the stress hormone, cortisol, in your body.

Estimated time: 50 minutes (including waiting time)

½ cup magnesium flakes

¼ cup coconut oil

3 tbsp. Shea butter

2 tbsp. beeswax pastilles

1. Place the magnesium flakes in a small bowl and drop 3 tbsp. of boiling water in it. Stir the mixture to melt the flakes in water. Set side.

2. Meanwhile, place all the remaining ingredients in a glass bowl Melt and stir everything by placing the bowl on top of simmer water.

3. Remove the bowl from the heat and allow the mixture to cool at room temperature.

4. When the mixture has cooled, grab a hand-held mixture and whip the mixture to create a

fully texture. While doing this, gradually add the melted magnesium flakes one drop at a time.

5. Continue blending until all the magnesium is incorporated in the mixture.

6. Transfer the body butter in the fridge to chill for 30 minutes and then whisk again before transferring into a sterilized container with a lid.

Goodbye Varicose! Body Butter

Are you losing your battle against those nasty varicose veins? Worry no more! This recipe combines essential oils that have muscle-relaxing and stress-relieving agents that also help reduce varicose veins

Estimated time: 2.5 hours (including waiting time)

½ cup Shea butter

¼ cup coconut oil

¼ cup jojoba oil

1 tbsp. vitamin E oil

10 drops lemon essential oil

10 drops cypress essential oil

10 drops fennel essential oil

1. Simmer water in a pot over low fire.

2. Place the coconut oil and Shea butter in a glass bowl and place on top of the pot with simmering water. Melt the ingredients together while stirring occasionally.

3. After the mixture has melted, remove the bowl from the heat and immediately pour in the

jojoba oil, lemon, cypress, fennel and Vitamin E oils. Combine well.

4. Place the bowl in the fridge to cool for 2 hours.

5. After 2 hours, use a hand-held blender to whip the mixture for 10 minutes or until you achieve a butter-like texture.

6. Store in an airtight container.

7. When applying this body butter recipe, begin from your ankles working your way upwards.

Calming Fruit Combo Body Butter

This is another body butter recipe that's sweet, aromatic, and calming that you surely would love to always use.

Estimated time: 50 minutes (including waiting time)

½ cup apricot kernel oil

5 drops orange essential oil

1 tsp. vitamin E oil

¼ cup cocoa butter

¼ cup Shea butter

1. Place the cocoa butter and Shea butter in a glass bowl and melt on top of a pot with simmering water. Stir occasionally.

2. Remove the bowl from the heat once the mixture has melted.

3. Immediately add the apricot oil, stir, and then transfer the bowl in the fridge to cool down for 30 minutes.

4. After 30 minutes, add the vitamin E oil and orange essential oil to the mixture.

5. Whip the body butter using a hand mixture until you achieve a fluffy texture.

6. Transfer the mixture into a container with a lid and store in a cool and dry area.

Jasmine Oil and Green Tea Infused Body Butter

Enjoy the health benefits of green tea, plus the calming effects of jasmine oil with this body butter recipe.

Estimated time: 50 minutes

1 teabag green tea

15 drops jasmine essential oil

1 ½ cups Shea butter

1 tsp. vitamin E oil

¾ cups olive oil

1. Melt the Shea butter in a glass bowl heated on top of a simmering pot of water.

2. Remove the bowl from the heat once the butter is completely melted.

3. Add the olive oil in the mixture along with the contents of the tea bag. Combine all the ingredients well.

4. Set aside the mixture and allow it to cool at room temperature for 15 minutes and then

transfer in the fridge to chill for another 15 minutes.

5. Remove the mixture from the fridge and then finally add the vitamin E oil along with the jasmine essential oil. Whisk using a hand-held mixture until you achieve a fully texture.

6. Store in an airtight container.

Aromatic Coffee Bar

Can't get enough of coffee? Here's a recipe caffeine addicts will surely love using!

Estimated time: 50 minutes (including waiting time)

¼ cup coconut oil infused with coffee

(just combine ½ cup coconut oil and 4 tbsp. ground coffee,

and then strain using a cheesecloth)

1 tbsp. beeswax

¼ cup cocoa butter

½ tsp. cocoa powder

½ tsp. cornstarch

1/8 tsp. cinnamon

1. Place the first three ingredients together in a glass blow.

2. Place the bowl on top of a pot of simmering water and melt the ingredients together, stirring occasionally.

3. When the mixture has completely melted, remove from heat and then add the remaining three ingredients. Combine well.

4. While the mixture is hot, pour it over small muffin tins.

5. Allow the mixture to harden into bars before storing in an airtight container.

Soothing Eucalyptus Body Butter

Proven to provide a soothing and calming effect, the eucalyptus essential oil stars in this body butter recipe which you will love using when you want relief from stress.

Estimated time: 1 hour (including waiting time)

12 drops eucalyptus essential oil

(you can also use peppermint)

2 ½ tbsp. olive oil

½ cup coconut oil

6 tbsp. Shea butter

6 tbsp. cocoa butter

1. Soften the cocoa butter, Shea butter, and coconut oil in a glass bowl placed on top of a pot of simmering water.

2. Remove the bowl from the heat and then add the olive oil and the eucalyptus essential oil. Mix well.

3. Chill the mixture in the fridge for 45 minutes or until the mixture is almost set.

4. After 45 minutes, whip the mixture using a hand-held blender and then mix until you achieve a fluffy texture.

5. Transfer in an air tight container and store in a cool and dry area.

Whipped Choco Body Butter

Who says chocolates are only for dessert? Here's an all-natural body butter recipe made with your favorite indulgence—chocolate! Make sure to control yourself not to eat it!

Estimated time: 50 minutes

2 tbsp. cocoa powder

½ cup cocoa butter

½ cup coconut oil

1. Place the coconut oil and cocoa butter in a glass bowl and melt over simmering pot of water.

2. Remove the bowl from the heat and place in the fridge for about 30-40 minutes, or until the mixture is almost set.

3. Using a hand-held mixer, whip the body butter until you achieve a fully texture.

4. Finally, add the cocoa powder to the mixture and combine until everything is well incorporated.

5. Store in an airtight sterilized jar. (This recipe can be stored up to 6 months.)

Matcha and Mint Body Butter

This recipe contains vegetable glycerin that contains an agent that helps protect your skin from bacteria.

Estimated time: 1.5 hrs. (including waiting time)

½ tbsp. matcha powder

8 pcs. mint leaves, chopped

½ cup Shea butter

½ cup coconut oil

1 tsp. olive oil

3 drops peppermint oil

1   tsp. vitamin E oil

1.   Melt the Shea butter along with the coconut oil in a glass bowl over a simmering pot of water. Stir occasionally.

2.   Once the mixture has melted, remove from the heat and chill in the fridge for about 30 minutes.

3. Remove the mixture from the fridge and then whip on high speed for 5 minutes or until the texture turns light and fluffy.

4. Place the bowl back in the fridge to allow to set for 15 minutes.

5. Once almost set, whip the mixture again and now gradually adding the peppermint oil.

6. Continue whisking for 5 minutes while adding the matcha powder, mint leaves and vitamin E oil.

7. Transfer in an airtight container. You can store this in the fridge up to 2 months.

All-in-One Healing Body Butter Mix

Can't find a solution for your stretch marks, scars, and other skin issues you can't hide? Give this body butter recipe a try and see those ugly marks disappear overtime.

Estimated time: 50 minutes

1 tsp. Argan oil

2 tsps. rosehip oil

15 drops vanilla extract

10 drops frankincense

½ cup cocoa butter

½ cup Shea butter

1. Melt the cocoa butter and Shea butter in a glass bowl placed on top of a simmering pot of water. Stir occasionally.

2. When the mixture has melted, remove the bowl from the heat and then add the remaining ingredients.

3. Place in the fridge to cool for 30 minutes and then whip the body butter using a hand-held mixer.

4. Transfer in an airtight container and store in a cool and dry area.

Whipped Vanilla Body Butter

Deeply moisturize your skin with this simple, yet delicious smelling body butter recipe.

Estimated time: 15 minutes

45 drops vanilla essential oil

1 cup Shea butter

½ cup coconut oil

1 tsp. vitamin E oil

1. Place all the ingredients in a glass bowl and combine them together using a hand-held mixture.

2. Whip the mixture for about 5 minutes or until you achieve a light and fluffy consistency.

3. Transfer in a jar with a lid and store in a cool and dry area.

Choco-Mint Body Butter

Chocolate and mint, how can you not fall in love with this recipe? Moisturize and refresh your skin with this body butter recipe, perfect for humid weather.

Estimated time: 15 minutes

30 drops peppermint essential oil

½ cup cocoa butter

½ cup coconut oil

4 tsp. cocoa powder

1. Combine the cocoa butter and coconut oil in a glass bowl and whisk them together using a hand-held mixture.

2. While whisking, gradually add the peppermint essential oil a few drops at a time.

3. When you almost achieve a fluffy texture, add in the cocoa powder, and then mix again for about 2 minutes.

4. Transfer the mixture into a container with a lid and store in a cool and dry area.

Honey and Lime Body Butter

Don't have much time to shop for ingredients for another homemade body butter? Here's a recipe using two pantry stapes—honey and lime.

Estimated time: 40 minutes (including waiting time)

10 drops lime essential oil

2 tbsp. beeswax

¼ tsp. vitamin E oil

½ cup grapeseed oil

2 tbsp. distilled water

1. Place the beeswax, vitamin E oil, and grapeseed oil in a glass bowl. Melt the mixture by placing the bowl on top of a simmering pot of water. Stir occasionally.

2. Remove the bowl from the heat once melted and then whip the mixture using a hand-held mixture on high speed.

3. Gradually add the water into the mixture, a few drops at a time, and continue to whip for a

few minutes until you achieve a light and airy texture.

4. Add the lime essential oil to the mixture and whip again.

5. Allow to sit for 15 minutes before transferring into your desired container.

Mango-Cookie Body Butter

Can't get enough of a "dessert-inspired" body butter recipe? Here's another one you can make at home!

Estimated time: 50 minutes (including waiting time)

½ cup cocoa butter

½ cup Shea butter

½ cup mango butter

3 tbsp. Argan oil

3½ tbsp. coconut oil

1 tsp. vitamin E oil

1/3 tbsp. sugar cookies fragrance oil

1. Place the cocoa butter, Shea butter, mango butter, and coconut oil in a glass bowl.

2. Melt the mixture by placing it on top of a simmering pot of hot water. Stir occasionally.

3. Once the mixture has melted and well incorporated, remove the bowl from the heat, and add the vitamin E and sugar cookies fragrance oil. Mix well.

4. Transfer the bowl in the fridge to cool and set for 30 minutes.

5. After 3 minutes, whip the mixture using a hand-held blender until you achieve an airy and light consistency.

6. Transfer the body butter in an airtight container.

Calm-Inducing Body Butter

This simple body butter recipe is the one you want to lather on your skin after a stressful day at work.

Estimated time: 40 minutes

¾ cup coconut oil

¼ cup cocoa butter

10 drops lavender essential oil

1. Combine the first two ingredients together in a glass bowl.

2. Melt them by placing the bowl on top of a simmering pot of water. Stir occasionally.

3. Once melted, remove the bowl from the heat and place in the fridge to cool for at least 30 minutes, or until the top is turning opaque.

4. Remove from the fridge and then whip using a hand-held mixture for while adding the lavender drops gradually. Whip until you achieve an airy consistency.

The Minimalist Body Butter

Are you left with only coconut oil and cocoa butter in your stash? No worries! You can still turn these two ingredients to a moisturizing body butter.

Estimated time: 50 minutes

¾ cup coconut oil

¼ cup cocoa butter

1. Place the two ingredients together in a glass bowl.

2. Melt them, but not boil, by placing the bowl on top of a simmering pot of water.

3. Once melted, remove the bowl from the heat and place in the fridge to cool for at least 30 minutes, or until the top is turning opaque.

4. Remove from the fridge and then whip using a hand-held mixture for about 5-7 minutes, or until you achieve a butter-like texture.

Body Scrub and Mask Recipes

Simple Sugar Scrub – Your Way

Use this easy recipe to create a basic sugar scrub in your favorite scent. Get zesty with some lemon, or sooth away your day with the scent of lavender.

Estimated time: 5 minutes or less

3 tablespoons granulated sugar

1 tablespoon of olive oil

15-20 drops of your favorite essential oil

1. Mix the ingredients together.
2. Rub mixture on your body and then rinse.

Banana Foster Body Scrub

This oil-free body scrub does your body good. The beneficial nutrients of the banana will leave your skin soft and glowing...it tastes delicious too!

Estimated time: 5 minutes

1 ripe banana

3 tablespoons granulated sugar

¼ teaspoon pure vanilla extract

1. Smash ingredients together with a fork. Don't over-mash or it will become too thin.

2. Pat the sugar mixture onto your body and gently massage it into your skin.

3. For your face, gently massage plain banana there, avoiding the eye area.

4. Rinse off with warm water.

Rosemary Lemon Salt Scrub

The aroma of rosemary and lemon will leave you feeling fresh and lively. Use this scrub to spruce up your shower.

Estimated time: 5 minutes

1 cup kosher salt

1/2 cup of pure organic almond oil

The zest of one lemon

2 teaspoons of fresh rosemary leaves

1. Pour the salt into a clean, sterilized container with a tight-fitting lid.

2. Add the lemon zest and rosemary.

3. Pour the almond oil over top and screw the lid on tightly.

4. Before using, give the jar a stir to mix the oil and salt together and then scrub away!

Skin Protecting Tomato Scrub

The natural antioxidants found in a tomato will protect your skin and slow down the effects of aging. This easily absorbable scrub will enhance your inner beauty!

Estimated time: 10 minutes

One ripe and organic tomato

Cutting knife

1 tablespoon of fine granulated sugar

1. Cut off the top of the tomato and cover it with the sugar.

2. Use the sugar-coated tomato top to exfoliate your face, especially your nose and forehead.

3. Wait 10 minutes and then rinse off the scrub.

4. Add the left-over tomato to your next meal!

Yummy Vanilla Coconut Brown Sugar Scrub

This scrub can double as dessert! The coconut oil is super moisturizing and fragrant. You will think you're in the tropics when using this one!

Estimated time: 5 minutes

1/2 cup coconut oil

1/2 cup brown sugar

1/2 teaspoon vanilla extract

1. Mix the ingredients together in a bowl or jar.

2. Rub the mixture on your skin while in the shower.

3. Massage the scrub into your skin and then rinse.

Sleepy Lavender Salt Scrub

This soothing scrub will release your body of dead skin and leave you calm and glowing.

Estimated time: 5 minutes

1/2 cub of coarse sea salt

1/3 cup of coconut oil

1 tablespoon of dried lavender

16 drops of lavender essential oil

1. Mix the salt and coconut oil together in a bowl or jar.
2. Add in the dried lavender and lavender oil.
3. Mix it all up and start scrubbing!

Homemade Apple Cider Facial Mask

This mask is particularly beneficial for oily skin. It leaves your face feeling super fresh and clean, with a nice tingly sensation.

Estimated time: 10 minutes

1/4 cup of Apple Cider Vinegar

1/2 cup water

1/2 cup of salt

1. Mix the ingredients together and wash it over your face.

2. Let the mixture dry on your face and leave it on for about 10 minutes, then rinse.

Going Green Avocado Facial Mask

Estimated time: 15 minutes

1 avocado

1 teaspoon of lemon juice

1 teaspoon of olive oil

1 teaspoon of honey

1. Remove the pit of the avocado and mash it until it has a smooth consistency.

2. Add the lemon, olive oil, and honey and mix.

3. Apply a thin layer of the mixture to your face and gently rub it in.

4. Let it sit for 15 minutes, then rinse.

Morning Coffee Facial Scrub

The coffee in this scrub will exfoliate your skin while the olive oil provides moisture and hydration – it's the best of both worlds!

Estimated time: 5 minutes or less

4 tablespoons of olive oil

6 tablespoons of fine coffee grounds

1. Mix the coffee grounds and olive oil until the scrub looks like coarse mud.
2. Scrub the mixture onto your skin and then rinse.

Cinnamon Exfoliating Scrub

Remove dead skin cells and rejuvenate your skin using this simple scrub recipe.

Estimated time: 5 minutes or less

1 cup lightly packed brown sugar

½ cup coconut oil

1 tsp. vitamin E oil

½ tsp. cinnamon powder

1. Combine all the ingredients in a food processor and pulse until the ingredients are well incorporated.

2. Damped your skin with water before massaging this mixture on your skin for 2 minutes. Rinse with warm water.

Sweet and Citrusy Body Scrub

This recipe contains olive oil which helps protect your skin from the harmful rays of the suns as well as clearing your skin with harmful toxins.

Estimated time: 5 minutes or less

1 cup brown sugar

1 tsp. vitamin E oil

½ cup olive oil

grapefruit drops lemon or lime extract

1. Combine all the ingredients in a food processor and pulse until the ingredients are well incorporated.

2. Dampen your skin with water before massaging this mixture on your skin for 2-3 minutes. Rinse with warm water.

Matcha Body Scrub

We all know that matcha, or green tea a number of benefits for the body, including the skin. Try this out this recipe for your homemade body scrub.

Estimated time: 5 minutes or less

3 cups Epsom salt

4 tbsp. sweet almond oil

3 tbsp. baking soda

1 tbsp. matcha powder

16 drops lime essential oil

1 zest of lime

1. Mix the baking soda, sweet almond oil, lime essential oil and salt in a bowl.

2. Add the matcha powder along with the lime zest and stir well.

3. Store in an airtight container.

Mango Mix Body Scrub

Try out this delicious smelling scrub during your bath time.

Estimated time: 5 minutes or less

½ cup sugar

3 tbsp. coconut oil (melted)

4 drops orange essential oil

¼ cup ripe mango, chopped

1. Place all the ingredients in a mixing bowl and mash everything together to incorporate.

2. Use this mixture to massage your body. Rinse thoroughly.

Olive Oil and Salt Scrub

Creating your homemade body scrub don' always mean you have to go shop for ingredients. This recipe uses two basic kitchen ingredients—olive oil and sea sat

Estimated time: 5 minutes or less

½ cup olive oil

½ cup sea salt

1. Combine the two ingredients in a mixing bowl and allow to sit for a few minutes.

2. Use this mixture as a scrub on your body. Rinse with cold water and then warm water after. Don't forget to pat dry your skin and then moisturize after.

Oats and Tea Body Scrub

Oats and tea aren't just for breakfast! You can also use them for your exfoliating baths.

Estimated time: 5 minutes or less

1 cup oats

4 tbsp. chamomile tea

(just remove contents from teabag)

½ cup grapeseed oil

½ cup coconut oil (melted)

1. Place the oats in a food processor and pulse until they are finely chopped.

2. Transfer the chopped oats in a mixing bowl and add the remaining ingredients.

3. Use this scrub recipe at the end of your shower routine. Allow the mixture to stay on your skin for a few minutes before rinsing thoroughly.

Honey and Oatmeal Autumn Facial Scrub:

Estimated time: 5 minutes

1/2 cup of oatmeal

2 tablespoons of organic honey

1 tablespoon nutmeg

15 drops of Lavender essential oil 15 drops of Tea Tree essential oil

1. Run oatmeal through the blender or food processor to break it up a bit.
2. Transfer the oatmeal into a bowl or jar and add the remaining ingredients.
3. Scrub the mixture on your body in the shower and then rinse.

The Health Benefits of Your Ingredients

Use this helpful table to compare the health benefits of all the ingredients used in this book's recipes – it will help you decide what to use when trying to create your own recipes! I hope this book leaves you with the knowledge you need to become a master butter or scrub maker, and as always, practice makes perfect!

Ingredient	Health Benefits
Olive Oil	Gentle moisturizing, helps skin irritations such as eczema and psoriasis, leaves skin feeling and looking youthful.
Banana	Slows down the proliferation of unwelcome wrinkles, hydrates skin, guards skin against bacteria, fades dark spots and blemishes, lightens skin tone, fights free radicals, enhances skin's UV resistance.
Vanilla	Relaxing and pleasing affect on the body, mind and spirit,

used as an aphrodisiac.

Lemon	Diminishes scars and age spots, heals acne, exfoliates, brightens and lightens skin, tones oily skin and fights wrinkles.
Rosemary	Supports healthy collagen development, contains antioxidants, good source of iron, calcium and vitamin B6.
Almond Oil	Anti-inflammatory, antiviral, antibacterial, and antiseptic properties.
Tomato	Antioxidants, projects skin against U.V rays, and slows down the affects of aging.
Coconut Oil	Strengthens underlying tissue, removes dead skin cells, antibacterial, antiviral, anti-fungal, contains antioxidants.
Lavender Oil	Anti-inflammatory, antioxidant, antiseptic, anti-fungal properties, soothes

	agitated skin, has a calming and pleasant scent.
Brown Sugar	Exfoliant, sloughs off dead surface skin, and reveals a new layer of healthy youthful skin, soothing and grounding fragrance.
Granulated Sugar	Exfoliant, sloughs off dead surface skin, and reveals a new layer of healthy youthful skin.
Coarse Salt	Exfoliant, sloughs off dead surface skin, and reveals a new layer of healthy youthful skin.
Oatmeal	Exfoliant, amino acids, hypoallergenic and moisturizing.
Honey	Reduces breakouts, moisturizing properties, antiseptic qualities that can reduce scars and encourage wound healing.

Nutmeg	Astringent, antibacterial, and anti-inflammatory properties.
Tea Tree Oil	Antibacterial, anti-inflammatory, antioxidant, antiseptic, immune stimulant properties, can heal and prevent acne.
Apple Cider Vinegar	Can kill pathogens, including bacteria, can clear skin problems and stop acne, anti-fungal, high levels of vitamins.
Avocado	Moisturizing, contains vitamins A, D and E, able to penetrate the skin, soothes sunburned skin, can boost collagen production and treat age spots, can reduce inflammation of the skin.
Coffee	Exfoliant, sloughs off dead surface skin, pick-me-up.
Shea Butter	Moisturizing, may help heal burns, sores, scars, dermatitis, psoriasis, may diminish

wrinkles.

Vitamin E Oil	Promotes healing, strong antioxidant that prevents premature aging.
Jojoba Oil	Moisturizing, reduces skin inflammation, fights against acne.
Cocoa and Mango Butter	Moisturizing agents, quickly absorbs into the skin, penetrates into your skin so that the body is able to retain the moisture.
Kukui Nut Oil	Leaves the skin feelings silky and smooth. Contains vitamins A, C, and E, which are antioxidants.

Conclusion

Congrats! You made it through the book! Hopefully you have a solid understanding now of how you can treat your skin and body with all natural ingredients from nature... And hopefully you don't go back to the old ways of store bought! (Unless it's organic and natural) ☺

Book 2:
Homemade Soap Making

Homemade Soap for Beginners - The Complete Guide to Making Luxurious, Skin-Softening Soap at Home

Karen Wells

Table of Contents

Introduction

Making soap at home may seem daunting, but there's no need to worry. All the basics you need to know about making your own soap are contained within these pages. This book is intended for complete beginners, though those already familiar with creating soap will learn new things too.

This book has everything from why you should make your own soap, to the history of soap making, to all you need to know to make your own soap. You'll learn the basics of soap making and even learn some beginner recipes for you to try, including guidelines to creating your own recipes! Learn about cold vs. hot process soap making, the nourishing health benefits of using natural soap ingredients, and all necessary safety precautions you'll need to take.

Once you've read the last page of this book on creating soap, you will be able to walk away with the knowledge you need to make your own bars of soap with confidence and ease. Share your knowledge with your friends, or even host a soap-making party!

Why You Should Toss Your Commercially-Produced Soaps

On an average day, people wash their hands an astounding 7-10 times! Though the blanket term of "soap" is applied to all sorts of things from the soaps used for dishes for the soaps used for cars, not all soap is composed of the same thing. The brightly colored soaps lining supermarket shelves have little in common with traditional soap. Though commercial soap has a bright and often delicious-smelling covering, these trappings are covering something quite different from the soap your grandmother used to use.

Commercially produced soaps both liquid and solid often contain artificial lathering agents, artificial colors, and countless unpronounceable chemicals—some of which can actually be quite harmful. For example, take triclosan, an antibacterial agent in many of the most popular soaps on the market. According to scientists, triclosan can increase bacterial and antibiotic resistance, cause skin irritation, and can even disrupt the metabolism. Other popular soap ingredients like pthalates and parabens can cause reproductive disorders and cancers.

It is tempting to drive to the store and buy soap. Commercial soaps are constantly marketed to keep consumers buying. Nevertheless, good marketing isn't always a good thing. Compare fast food companies marketing their unhealthy foods to commercial soap companies marketing their chemical-laden soaps. You know that these products aren't what are best for your body and that it's better to make them yourself!

The Wondrous Benefits of Making Your Own Soap!

Check the label on the soaps in your bathroom. How many of the ingredients can you comfortably identify? Triclosan, sodium laureth sulfate, methylparaben... The list goes on. Imagine what it would be like to know exactly what's in your soap by making it yourself!

Did you know that glycerin, which used to be an essential aspect of traditional soap, is separated out by commercial soap producers and resold to be included in more expensive beauty products? Natural handmade soap bars retain all of the good ingredients to moisturize your skin the natural way.

Creating your own soap, full of incredible essential oils and natural oils and fats to moisturize your skin, is not only fun but also good for your body. You will gain peace of mind knowing exactly what you're using on your skin. You can even gain more peace of mind from putting the right essential oils in your soap! Lavender, a classic soap ingredient, can relieve nervous tension, relieve pain, disinfect, and enhance blood circulation. Lavender's Latin name is Lavare, which means "to wash," no doubt due to its clean, fresh aroma. Blend lavender with other essential oils like cedarwood or pine to personalize your soap's scent and of course, its health benefits.

Not only is making your own soap good for you (not to mention an enjoyable hobby), but it is also extremely cost efficient. Making homemade soap takes more time than going to the store, but the results are certainly worth the extra effort. For most basic soaps, you simply need just four core ingredients: water, oil or fat, antioxidants, and lye, all of which can be easily acquired to make enough soap to give out as presents over the holidays!

Common Myths about Homemade Soap Making

1. It's too expensive.

Though the initial shopping trip for ingredients may be daunting, homemade soap is actually quite reasonable. One savvy soap maker calculated costs for basic unscented (and of course, homemade) soap at 15 cents per ounce of soap. Of course, purchasing ingredients in larger quantities will be more cost effective. Essential oils for fragrance can sometimes be pricy, so keep an eye out for deals online and in health food stores.

2. It's too difficult.

If you can measure ingredients, you can make soap! Making soap might have been very time consuming and difficult in your grandmother's time, but with today's modern tools, making soap can be about as simple as making a cake. A digital scale and immersion blender, though not essential for making soap, will definitely be an asset in your soap making process.

3. It's too dangerous.

Lye does seem like an intimidating ingredient, and you may have concerns over the need to use lye in your soap. As long as you are careful, there is nothing to fear. The lye reacts with oil in a process called saponification, and if you measure correctly, then there will be no lye in your final homemade soap. Just be sure to use glasses or goggles and kitchen rubber gloves to protect your eyes and skin from becoming irritated by the lye.

What Is Soap Making, Anyway?

Soap Making Overview

People have been making soap for thousands upon thousands of years. Ancient Romans are often credited with the discovery of soap, with the legend telling of fat dripping off an animal sacrifice, mixing with the ashes of the fire below it, and that mixture making its way to a river where women found their laundry much easier to clean with the substance. The hill the women were on was called Sapo, so the concoction was said to be named after the hill! Evidence has been found, however, of earlier soap making across the world.

Ingredients for soap making were commonly found from both animal and vegetable sources. Ancient Celts, for example, made their soap from animal fat and plant ashes, naming their product "saipo," from which our modern word soap may also be derived!

The first to produce soaps from vegetable oils and aromatic oils were Arabic chemists. These chemists produced perfumed and even colored soaps.

Soaps were primarily homemade or artisanal until approximately the eighteenth century. As medical science developed, the role of hygiene and the understanding of the relationship between cleanliness and health grew and popularized the concept of industrially produced bar soaps became readily available.

Commercial soap, as we know it today, came after the end of the First World War. Today, the soap industry is booming. What many people do not know about commercial soap is that similar methods of production are used today as were the 1800's!

The cold process method is most popular with modern soap makers, though some soap makers use the more historical hot process. Cold process soap is made from specific proportions of fats or oils and lye in a process called saponification, which occurs with very little heat. Soap produced by the cold process method takes approximately six weeks to be completely ready for use and can last for a long time.

Hot process soap, however, is a different take than the cold process method. In a contrast to cold process, hot process soap does not require as much scientific measuring. All the ingredients for the soap are put into a pot over a heat source and stirred continuously until all excess water has evaporated. The soap is then ready to use because of the higher temperature enabling quicker saponification!

Basic Soap Making Terms to Know

Acid
See "fatty acid"

Alkali
A compound with a pH greater than 7, also known as a base. Some examples include Sodium Hydroxide (lye) and Potassium Hydroxide.

Antioxidant
A substance that slows or prevents oxidation and helps prevent spoilage in soap.

Base
See "alkali."

Botanical
Related to plants or plant life.

Castile Soap
A soap made with a high percentage of olive oil, named for its origins in a region in Spain.

Caustic
Able to burn or corrode. Lye is also known as caustic soda.

Cold Process
A method of soap making that requires heat to melt oils but no direct cooking.

Cure
The time period between making the soap and using it.

Cold process soap should be left for 4-6 weeks before its use to allow for the soap to completely saponify.

Detergent
A cleansing substance that acts similarly to soap, but is made from chemicals rather than fats and lye.

Emollient
Used to soften, smooth, and moisturize the skin, emollients are often vegetable oils and glycerin.

Essential Oil
A plant-based oil that has been harvested for its odor, flavor, or healthful benefits.

Exfoliant
An ingredient added to soap to help slough dead skin cells and dirt from the skin.

Fatty Acids
These compounds found in fats and oils give soap their lather, hardness, cleansing, and conditioning characteristics.

Fragrance Oil
Synthetic scented oil used instead of essential oil.

Gel Stage
A stage of soap making once it has been poured into the mold and becomes translucent.

Glycerin
A thick, sticky, and clear substance created during saponification, glycerin is also a natural emollient.

Hot Process
A method of soap making that requires external heat to cause quicker saponification.

Irritant
Substance that can cause inflammation or a painful reaction on the skin.

Lard
Fat that has been rendered from animals, often pigs.

Lye
Also known as Sodium Hydroxide, this is an essential ingredient in the soap making process.

Melting Point
The temperature at which oil for soap making melts.

pH
The measure of acidity or alkalinity of a solution. A substance with pH greater than 7.0 is a base, and less than 7.0 is an acid. 7.0 is neutral.

Preservative
A natural or manufactured chemical that is added to prevent spoilage.

Saponification
The chemical reaction between lye and a fat or oil to form soap.

Seize
Too quickly solidifying soap while still in the soap pan, seizing is caused by the soap mixture having too much fat

with high amounts of certain acids or some fragrance and essential oils.

Soap
The result of a chemical reaction between lye and fats or oils. If it's not made with lye, it's not soap!

Soda Ash
White powder that can form on top of curing soap.

Superfatted
The excess oils left unsaponified in finished soap that contribute to moisturizing qualities of the soap.

Tallow
The fatty tissue of animals.

Trace
The soap is ready at the trace stage, when soap spooned from the mixture and drizzled on top floats on top of the solution for a short while before sinking back down.

Basic Equipment and Ingredients Needed

INGREDIENTS

Antioxidant

Antioxidants are an optional ingredient that will extend the life of your soap. I'd recommend rosemary oleoresin extract.

Crock Pot

A crock pot is handy when making hot process soap. A double boiler method also works well for this method, so use whatever is convenient.

Oils

Different oils have different effects on your soap. Olive oil and shea butter are moisturizing, coconut oil has good lather, and palm oil creates a firm bar. There are a few other oils, but these are the most basic that you'll be using in your first soaps. Most homemade soaps will contain a combination of oils, so it's best to follow a recipe first before experimenting with your own different proportions of oils.

Lye

Also known as sodium hydroxide, lye is what makes soap, soap! You can purchase lye from some supermarkets and hardware stores, but it has become increasingly difficult to find. Most lye is not labeled for soap making and is instead used as a drain cleaner. Make sure that if you do find lye from these sources that it is 100% sodium hydroxide! Buying lye online for soap making is also a great option.

Scent

You can choose to leave your soap unscented, or you can add small quantities of essential oils or fragrance oils to scent your home made soap.

Water

Water plays an important role in the chemical processing of lye. Make sure that you don't use hard water for cold process soap making, as some of the minerals could react with the lye. I recommend using distilled water.

EQUIPMENT

Immersion blender

An immersion blender, also known as a stick blender, will ensure a smooth and consistent result. An immersion blender is not required, but will turn strenuous stirring into a few minutes' work.

Scale

It is important to measure all of your ingredients by weight, especially for small batches of soap. Digital scales are easy to read and can be used for precise baking.

Stainless Steel Pot

Lye will react with a cast iron, nonstick, or aluminum pot, so make sure to use a stainless steel or enamel-covered pot for making your soap.

Bowls/Containers

It's always helpful to have a variety of bowls and containers for both measuring and mixing. At least one of these bowls should be heat resistant for working with hot materials, so look for a bowl that is stainless steel or pyrex. Don't forget that lye will react with aluminum! Do not use wood bowls, either. Wood can absorb dangerous chemicals.

Drying Rack

Drying racks are important to assist with airflow when soap is curing.

pH Testing Kit

You may want to test the pH of your earliest soaps to make sure they are not too basic.

Spoons

You'll want to have measuring spoons and mixing spoons on hand. Do not use a wooden spoon.

Thermometer

It's important to keep track of what temperature your soap mixture is to create the right balance in your soap. More than one thermometer will simplify your process. More on the two thermometers later!

Soap Mold

A soap mold can be any container. You can use a wood or plastic box, or even a milk carton! Soap molds in pretty shapes are also an option and can be purchased or made at home. I'll show you how to make some further on in the book.

Freezer Paper

Line your soap molds with freezer paper to prevent sticking.

Cardboard Box

If you can, find a box that is large enough to cover your soap mold.

Knife

Any old kitchen knife with a large blade will do the trick.

Glasses and Gloves

These two pieces of equipment are essential when dealing with lye. Handling lye is completely safe when done correctly, so be sure to wear rubber gloves to protect your hands and goggles or safety glasses to protect your eyes.

General Safety Guidelines

The importance of safety cannot be stressed enough when making soap. Though making soap at home can be easy and fun, working with chemicals and mixing ingredients over heat warrants some caution. Don't forget your gloves and goggles when you're dealing with lye, and be careful when handling hot ingredients and tools! It is also recommended to wear closed-toe shoes, and avoid a lot of exposed skin on your arms and legs. If you're making soap indoors, be sure to open a few windows to keep the room ventilated. You should also keep a bottle of vinegar handy in case you spill any lye, as it will neutralize the chemical.

Be sure to store your lye in an airtight container in a place you know children or pets cannot get into it. Also, make sure to store your soap in a safe place, as some soaps can look (and smell) tempting to pets and children.

Let's Prepare! How to Make Your Own Soap Molds

Purchasing soap molds can get expensive, and once you get the soap bug you'll likely want to spend your hard-earned money on fragrance oils and essential oils! The good news is that you don't have to spend a lot of money on soap molds. Here are a few tips for molding your soap that won't break the bank.

A great way to make round soap bars (hot process method only) is with cylindrical chip or oatmeal canisters. Clean the can out, spoon in the soap, and just tear the can off when you're ready to cut it!

I've found that yogurt containers can serve as great individual soap molds. Novelty silicone ice trays can make cute tiny soaps to pile up in a dish.

Another easy method of making your own soap molds is with milk cartons. Carefully cut the side off of a square half gallon of milk, clean it, and pour your soap in. There's no need to line the carton, as it is already lined in wax! A milk carton mold will hold approximately 2-3 pounds of soap.

If you want a bigger mold but don't want to go out and buy one, why not try a shoe box or cereal box? Be sure to line the mold with freezer paper.

Remember, you don't want your soap touching any metal besides stainless steel. Don't be afraid to get creative.

Look in the baking aisle for candy molds, loaf pans, and more to shape your soap.

If you're feeling particularly crafty, why not try to make your own soap mold? I'm all thumbs when it comes to woodcraft, but if you know your way around a drill, why not try to make your own soap mold out of wood?

Step-by-Step Cold Process Soap Making

Overview, Pros and Cons

The term "cold" is perhaps a misnomer, as cold process soap making actually involves a bit of heat! You'll be creating this heat through chemical reactions, and you'll need to melt solid fats before mixing them. Cold process soap making is a more modern way to make soap than the hot process, but it is definitely worth it.

Cold process soap is much faster to be poured into molds than hot process soap. This cold process does involve the need for very precise mixing, but the reward is that your soap will last (make it in large quantities!). This process also requires you to wait anywhere from three to eight weeks for your soap to cure. Cold process soap making creates soap that is harder and longer lasting than the hot process method.

Step by Step How-To

Estimated time: 1.5 hours

1. Gather your Supplies

Put on your rubber gloves and goggles! Keep them on until you are completely done with all of your soap making. Make sure you have all of the supplies you need for the recipe you're using. Refer to the equipment section to see exactly what you'll be using to make your soap.

2. Prep the Lye Mixture

Carefully weigh your lye according to your recipe. To avoid spilling lye all over your scale, you can use a container or a cup (don't forget to zero the scale after putting the container) to measure your lye. Try to make the measurements as exact as possible. Measure your water into a heat resistant vessel. The recipes here will tell you exactly how much water to use, but as a general rule you should use 3 ounces of water to every 1 ounce of lye. Remember, always pour the lye into the water and not the other way around! Mix continuously until the lye is completely dissolved. Be very careful when mixing, as the chemical reaction will increase the temperature of the mixture to over 200 degrees Fahrenheit. Measure the temperature of your mixture with a thermometer and set it aside in a safe area.

3. Prep the Fatty Acids

Pour the correct weights of the oils or fats into a large pot. The measuring of these ingredients must always be done by weight for the ideal soap making results. Liquids are fine to go straight into the pot, but solid fats or oils need a little more prep. Melt your solid fatty acids in a smaller saucepan on low heat until liquid, and then add these to the large pot. Once you get more experienced making soap, you can experiment with superfatting your soap (adding extra fat) for added skin benefits of these oils. You can also add a preservative (antioxidant) to the fats and oils at this point if you so desire. Put your second thermometer in this mixture and set it aside!

4. Wait and Adjust

Most soap recipes will tell you what temperature is ideal, but generally, you want your mixtures to be between 95 and 110 degrees Fahrenheit depending on what kind of soap you're making. Make sure both of your mixtures are around the same temperature when you mix them, but it's likely that you'll have to do some adjusting. You can either put the containers in cold water or hot water.

5. Mix

Pour the lye into the fatty acids. Stir the solution constantly and rapidly. You can either use a spoon to mix in a figure eight pattern or, for much faster results, use an immersion blender. You'll know when the mixture is ready when it starts to saponify. This stage is called trace. You can test this by spooning some soap onto the surface of the liquid. If it floats, your soap is ready! If not, keep mixing. Hand mixing can take forty five minutes to an hour to reach trace, but an immersion blender can decrease this time to as little as five minutes!

6. Customize

Add the other ingredients, such as essential oils, fragrance, dyes, or exfoliants. Mix until ingredients are evenly distributed.

7. Pour into Molds and Cover

Pour the soap into your choice of mold. You can use individual molds for individual soaps, or pour your soap into a larger mold and cut it into bars after it has hardened. Cover the mold with a lid or a piece of cardboard and wrap it with lots of towels or some other fabric. The mixture is continuing to saponify while it is in the molds. It will actually get hotter before cooling off! You don't want much heat to escape, as it is essential to the early curing process. Leave the soap for anywhere to 18-36 hours (depending on the recipe).

8. Cut and Cure your Soap

If you've made your soap in a large mold, you'll want to cut it once it's solidified and is hard enough to slice. Use a sharp knife to cut your soap into even slices. If you used individual molds, gently remove the soap from the molds.

Lay your soap on a drying rack. The soap will need to cure for three to eight weeks depending on the recipe. Rotate your soap every week! When the curing process is done, make sure to wipe off any soda powder that has formed, as it can be drying on the skin. For your first few batches, you may want to test the pH level with a kit to make sure your soap is completely saponified. If your strip reads between 7 and 10, the soap is no longer caustic and is safe to touch.

9. Clean Up

It's best to wash your tools by hand to avoid leftover soap from causing your dishwasher to leak! You probably won't want to cook with your soap making pots to avoid any chemical contamination.

20 Nourishing Cold Process Soap Recipes

Now it's your turn to make some soap! Use the cold-process soap making process you just learned about to make the below recipes – and remember, have fun!

All recipes will produce 5 pounds of soap. All weights are in ounces (by weight, not by volume unless for additives).

Recipes can be scaled down proportionally, but be careful with the math!
http://www.soapcalc.net/calc/SoapCalcWP.asp is a very helpful website that can not only assist you when making your own recipes, but can also help scale recipes down or up. This site is great for cold or hot process soap making.

Simply Soothing Soap

This is a no frills, uncomplicated recipe that you can tweak with different essential oils and colorants. One of the hardest parts of cold process soap making is recognizing trace. Test for trace frequently to make sure you don't miss it! If you keep stirring for too long, your soap will likely solidify in the pot. 26.5 ounces olive oil

16.5 ounces coconut oil

10 ounces palm oil

7.37 ounces lye

20 ounces distilled water

Temperature to adjust to ("wait and adjust"): 95 degrees

Insulation time: one full day

Curing time: 4-6 weeks

Luxurious Lavender Soap

This soap, which includes oats and lavender, is soothing for skin and helps provide an aromatherapy experience. This recipe is also 5% superfatted!

21.2 ounces olive oil

10.6 ounces palm oil

3.18 ounces shea butter

4.77 ounces rice bran oil

10.6 ounces coconut oil

2.65 ounces castor oil

2.65 ounces lavender oil

4 tablespoons colloidal oatmeal (finely ground whole oats)

20 ounces oat milk* (instead of water)

7.27 grams lye

Optional: lavender buds for decoration after pouring into molds

*How to make oat milk:

Mix one cup of whole oats (not quick oats) with three cups of water and blend on high until smooth. Strain over cheesecloth or a fine strainer.

Temperature to adjust to ("wait and adjust"): 110 degrees

Insulation time: one full day

Curing time: 6-8 weeks

Honey Oatmeal Soap

This soap smells delicious and includes therapeutic clove bud and sweet orange essential oils. You'll want to add your almond milk immediately after you pour the lye into your oils mixture so the mix doesn't get too thick. Stir manually for a few minutes, then go ahead and add the honey, then the oatmeal, then the essential oils.

26.5 ounces olive oil

10.6 ounces coconut oil

6.4 ounces sweet almond oil

5.3 ounces avocado oil

4.3 ounces castor oil

2.5 ounces honey diluted with 3 ounces of warm water

6 ounces almond milk

2 ounces whole oats (to sprinkle on top after pouring into mold)

1.59 ounces sweet orange essential oil

1.06 ounces clove bud essential oil

12 ounces water

7.28 ounces lye

Temperature to adjust to ("wait and adjust"): 80-90 degrees

Insulation time: one full day

Curing time: 6-8 weeks

Cup of Coffee Soap

This bar of soap won't wake you up in the morning quite as well as a cup of coffee, but its delicious aroma will make for the perfect morning shower. Do not add powdered cinnamon or nutmeg instead of essential oils to your mixture as they can irritate the skin!

23.85 ounces olive oil

8.5 ounces coconut oil

10.6 ounces palm oil

5.3 ounces rice bran oil

2.65 ounces sweet almond oil

2.1 ounces castor oil

1.34 ounces coffee essential oil

.332 ounces nutmeg essential oil

6 ounces strong brewed coffee, cooled (to be added with the essential oils in the "customize" step)

14 ounces water

7.2 ounces lye

Temperature to adjust to ("wait and adjust"): 90-100 degrees

Insulation time: 12-24 hours

Curing time: 6-8 weeks

Smooth as Silk Shaving Bar

You'll love the rich lather and protective layer this shaving bar will provide. Use with a shaving brush for luxurious results. Mix the bentonite clay in very slowly to prevent clumping. Add the bentonite clay first, then the oatmeal.

23.9 ounces olive oil

10.6 ounces coconut oil

10.6 ounces castor oil

4.2 ounces palm oil

3.7 ounces sweet almond oil

3 tablespoons bentonite clay

4 tablespoons colloidal oatmeal

20 ounces water

7.27 ounces lye

Temperature to adjust to ("wait and adjust"): 110 degrees

Insulation time: Do not insulate your soap to allow it to stay very creamy. Let it solidify for 12-24 hours.

Curing time: 4-6 weeks

2-Pound Batch Cold Process Soap Recipes

For readers who may not want to make as much as 5-pound batches, the following recipes are about 2 pounds each. These are perfect for a 10-inch loaf mold, making about 7-8 4-ounce bars. For cold process soaps, you will want your oils and lye mixture to cool to about 100-120F before mixing. Soaps should be insulated for 24-48 hours, and cure for 3-4 weeks before use (exclusive of Castile soap).

Pomegranate Exfoliation Bar

The super fruit pomegranate is also great for your skin, offering moisturizing, anti-oxidant, and anti-inflammatory properties. This simple recipe gives you extra exfoliating power with pomegranate powder.

7 ounces coconut oil

7 ounces olive oil

7 ounces vegetable shortening

3 ounces lye

6.8 ounces distilled water

1.6 ounces pomegranate fragrance oil

2 tbsp. pomegranate powder

red dye colorant

Add the pomegranate powder in the "Customize" step.

Ginger Lime Soap

The zing of sparkling ginger and fresh lime makes this bar the perfect morning pick-me-up soap. This recipe employs just an ounce of beeswax for additional hardness, ensuring that the bar will last longer.

1 ounce sweet almond oil

4 ounces canola oil

3 ounces castor oil

8 ounces coconut oil

3 ounces olive oil

3 ounces palm oil

1 ounce beeswax

7 ounces distilled water

3.24 ounces lye

1.4 ounce ginger lime fragrance oil

Yellow and green pigment-type colorant

In the "Customize" step, after adding your fragrance oil, divide the batch between two bowls, adding green colorant to one and yellow to the other. Pour the green into molds first and give it a minute or two to harden; then add the yellow to give your soap a layered look.

Bringin' Home the Bacon Lard Soap

Reminiscent of soaps of yore, this simple bar relies solely on lard for the fat content. Contrary to what some may believe, lard doesn't make soap greasy but is, in fact, mild, moisturizing and conditioning. For this novelty soap, I use bacon fragrance oil to really go whole hog.

22 ounces lard

8 ounces distilled water

2.84 ounces lye

1.2 ounces bacon fragrance oil

Mango Papaya Soap

This fruity soap smells good enough to eat! With an addition of castor oil and shea butter, this bar is both bubbly and silky. For this recipe I like to give the soap a pretty marbled effect using vibrant mica powder.

4 ounces castor oil

5 ounces coconut oil

5 ounces olive oil

3 ounces palm oil

3 ounces shea butter

2 ounces sweet almond oil

8 ounces distilled water

3 ounces lye

1.6 ounces mango papaya fragrance oil

½ tablespoon red-orange mica powder

In the "Customize" step, after adding your fragrance oil, divide the batch between two bowls. Blend the mica powder into one bowl. Pour the un-colored soap into your mold(s), followed by the red-orange soap. Using a skewer or butter knife, gently cut paths through the soap to swirl the colors, giving a beautiful marbled effect.

Lemongrass Green Tea Soap

Green tea is known to help prevent skin aging and has natural anti-inflammatory properties. Not only does this soap have a soothing scent, it employs dried lemongrass to gently exfoliate as you wash. If you can't find green tea butter, substitute with sweet almond oil.

2 ounces castor oil

8 ounces coconut oil

2 ounces green tea butter

4 ounces olive oil

16 ounces vegetable shortening

10 ounces strong brewed green tea

4.43 ounces lye

1.5 ounce lemongrass & green tea fragrance oil

.25 ounces lemongrass essential oil

2-4 tablespoons dried lemongrass

Stir in the dried lemongrass in the "Customize" stage. Save a little bit to sprinkle over your soap after you pour it into the mold(s).

Honey Apricot Soap

When used in just small amounts honey can greatly increase the benefits of your soap. Aside from giving your bar a nice moisturizing lather, it also has antimicrobial and anti-inflammatory properties that cleanse and soothe the skin.

4.4 ounces canola oil

5.5 ounces coconut oil

2.2 ounces jojoba oil

4.4 ounces olive oil

5.5 ounces palm oil

2 tbsp. honey

1.6 ounces honeyed apricot fragrance oil

Add the honey in the "Customize" step.

Goat's Milk & Honey Soap

Goat's milk has become a popular soap making base- and for a good reason. It contains alpha hydroxy acids that get rid of dead skin cells, a number of vitamins and minerals, moisturizing cream, and anti-bacterial properties. This bar is great for people with acne or other skin conditions.

1 ounce castor oil

5 ounces coconut oil

4.25 ounces olive oil

11 ounces vegetable shortening

3 ounces lye

12 ounces frozen, partially thawed goat milk

1.2 ounces Goat's Milk & Honey fragrance oil

2 tbsp. honey

Be sure to work slowly when adding lye to milk as it can scald easily and discolor your soap.

100% Castile

Castile soap gets its name from the Castile region of Spain, where bars of this hard olive-based soap have been made for hundreds of years. Bergamont essential oil adds a uplifting, mood enhancing appeal to this 100% olive oil soap. Be warned, this soap takes a lot of patience. For the best possible bar, you must wait at least 4 months for the soap to cure.

22 ounces olive oil

8 ounces distilled water

2.8 ounces lye

1.4 ounces bergamont essential oil

Nuts About Almond Soap

This soap recipe features almond, almond, and more almond in the form of oil, butter, and milk. I've also added a yummy almond fragrance oil to really make that warm, nutty scent pop. As opposed to a water base, the use of almond milk in this recipe adds extra skin nourishing benefits, but feel free to use water if you can't find any.

3 ounces almond butter

2 ounces sweet almond oil

2 ounces castor oil

6 ounces coconut oil

5 ounces olive oil

6 ounces vegetable shortening

6 ounces almond milk

3.3 ounces lye

1.4 ounces almond fragrance oil

Monkey Farts Soap for Kids

Don't let the name fool you, this combination of tropical fruits, banana and creamy coconut smells divine, and is especially popular with kids...or kids of all ages. The extra castor oil gives the soap a nice bubbly later, and the funky color blend makes this a soap that the young ones will love.

2.2 ounces canola oil

1.3 ounces castor oil

5.5 ounces coconut oil

5.5 ounces olive oil

5.5 ounces palm oil

2.2 ounces sunflower seed oil

7.3 ounces distilled water

3.1 ounces lye

1.7 ounces Monkey Farts fragrance oil

1 tsp. each hot pink, blue, and yellow oxide colorants

Before you begin, mix 1 tsp. of colorant with 1 tbsp. of olive oil in three separate bowls using a whisk or mini mixer. At trace, separate your soap into three bowls and add one mixed color to each. When you pour the soap into your molds, alternate colors and swirl.

Coconut Salt Scrub Bar

This tropical treat uses sea salt to gently exfoliate as you wash. Since the fats are 80% coconut oil it makes a nice hard bar. This soap is 50% salt, so it must be cut before completely set to avoid crumbling.

1.2 ounces avocado oil

2 ounces castor oil

12.8 ounces coconut oil

5.3 ounces coconut milk

2.4 ounces lye

16 ounces medium grain sea salt

1.6 ounces coconut fragrance oil

Before you begin, preheat the oven to 170F. Add the sea salt in the "Customize" step, and stir well before pouring into your mold. Place the mold in the heated oven and turn off the heat. Allow the soap to sit for about 2 hours until it is firm. Immediately cut into bars and set aside to cure.

Salted Caramel

Salted caramel is all the rage these days. Now you can rub the delicious aroma all over your skin! A small amount of fine sea salt adds to the longevity and cleansing power of the bar.

2 ounces castor oil

12 ounces coconut oil

4 ounces olive oil

2 ounces shea butter

2.89 ounces lye

6.6 ounces milk of your choice (cow, goat, almond, rice, whatever you have on hand!)

1.5 ounces caramel or salted caramel fragrance oil

7 ounces fine grain sea salt, 1 tbsp. reserved for topping

1 tsp. bronze mica powder

Add the salt and mica powder in the "Customize" step, blending thoroughly. After pouring into your mold, top with reserved salt.

The Bee's Knees Honeysuckle Soap

A little bit of beeswax goes a long way to contribute to the hardness of this bar. This floral soap will make you think of springtime, when the honeysuckle is just beginning to bloom. Place bubble wrap on top of your freshly poured soap to give it a neat honeycomb effect.

.42 ounces beeswax

1 ounce castor oil

5.9 ounces coconut oil

5.9 ounces olive oil

5.9 ounces palm oil

2.59 ounces lye

7 ounces water

1.3 ounces honeysuckle fragrance oil

2 tablespoons honey

Add honey in the "Customize" step.

Homemade Shampoo Bar

Homemade soap isn't just for your skin! This nifty shampoo bar uses castor and coconut oils for a nice bubbly lather, while sweet almond and jojoba oils help to condition your hair.

2.1 ounces canola oil

4.2 ounces castor oil

5.25 ounces coconut oil

1 ounce jojoba oil

4.2 ounces olive oil

2.1 ounces palm oil

2.1 ounces sweet almond oil

2.85 ounces lye

6.9 ounces water

1.5 ounces fragrance oil of choice- crisp apple, tropical coconut, and citrus splash are great options

Chocolate Lovers Soap

This delectable recipe triples up on the chocolate with cocoa butter for firmness and moisturizing qualities, cocoa powder for color, and chocolate fragrance oil for a strong, lasting scent. A chocoholic's dream!

2.2 ounces castor oil

2.2 ounces cocoa butter, non-deodorized

6.6 ounces coconut oil

6.6 ounces olive oil

4.4 ounces palm oil

3 ounces lye

7.26 ounces water

1.5 ounces chocolate fragrance oil

1 tbsp. cocoa powder

Add the cocoa powder in the "Customize" step.

Step-by-Step Hot Process Soap Making

Overview, Pros and Cons

Hot process soap making is very similar to cold process, but much of the mixing occurs either in a crock pot or over a double boiler. Soap made through this method tends to be fluffier than cold process soap, and it absorbs fragrance very effectively. A little goes a long way! Hot process soap allows you to use a wider range of colorants and additives that would otherwise react badly with the lye present in cold process soap making. Hot process soap can take more stirring and waiting than cold process soap, but the main benefit to this process is that your soap will be ready to use immediately after it has hardened. Hot process soap is more difficult to add designs to due to its texture when molding.

Step by Step How-To

Complete steps 1-3 from the cold process step by step instructions. Note: If you're using a crock pot, go ahead and melt your oils directly in the crock pot.

4. Mix

This is the main step that differentiates cold and hot process soap making! There is no need to wait for the oils and the lye mixture to reach the same temperature. Slowly pour the lye solution into your crock pot (set to medium) or into a double boiler and stir or use an immersion blender. Be careful when you're mixing not to splash, as the contents can be very hot. The mixture will begin to thicken in consistency and turn opaque. Keep stirring until it reaches trace.

5. Keep on Cooking!

Put the lid on your double boiler or crock pot and let your soap cook on low. Depending on the recipe, the cooking process can take anywhere from an hour to three hours. Check your soap occasionally, but don't stir it unless it looks like it's going to bubble over. While you're waiting, prep your colors and fragrances. If you notice the soap beginning to separate, stir it and put the lid back on. Once your soap has increased in volume, you'll want to keep stirring until it reaches the consistency of mashed potatoes. Turn off the crock pot or take the pot off the heat at this point. Keep stirring until you get soap that has the appearance of very thick, waxy mashed potatoes.

6. Personalize your Soap

Add your scents and colorants, and mix well.

7. Mold

Hot process soap does not pour like cold process soap. Instead, you'll need to carefully spoon it into your molds. Be as quick and careful as you can so that the mix doesn't cool down too quickly. You can smooth the top of the soap for a more consistent appearance with some parchment paper or leave the top rough for a different look. Gently tap your mold on the counter to release air bubbles.

8. Cut and Cure

Wait 48 hours for your soap to harden. If your soap is hard to remove from the mold, try putting it into the freezer for a short while. You can then cut your soap right away! Once you cut your hot process soap, you can either use it right away or let it cure for a few weeks for milder soap.

10 Fun Hot Process Soap Recipes

Again, use the hot process soap making technique you just learned about to make the below recipes. They smell amazing!

These recipes are designed to produce less soap than the cold process recipes, as the cooking process requires more room in the pot. Most recipes are between 2-3 pounds. All weights are in ounces (by weight, not by volume unless for additives).

Grapefruit Rosemary Soap

This recipe combines the citrusy scent of grapefruit with the fresh scent and health benefits of rosemary essential oil.

9.52 ounces coconut oil

12.699 ounces olive oil

9.52 ounces palm oil

11.5 ounces distilled water

4.43 ounces lye

1/8 tsp rosemary essential oil

1 teaspoon grapefruit fragrance oil

1 teaspoon sweet almond oil

Avocado Baby Soap

This soap is mild enough for a baby, and will be just as gentle and moisturizing on your skin. The last three ingredients (fragrance oil, vitamin E, and glycerin) should be added during the thin mashed potato stage. I like to dye this soap in pretty pastels.

12 ounces avocado oil

3 ounces coconut oil

9 ounces jojoba oil

2 ounces palm oil

2 ounces shea butter

10 ounces distilled water

3 ounces lye

1 tablespoon vanilla fragrance oil

1 teaspoon vitamin E

1 teaspoon glycerin

Candy Cane Soap

You'll love the pretty swirls and the peppermint fragrance of this candy cane soap. Remove a cup or so of the soap and dye it with the red colorant, then add it back in and stir gently.

2 ounces castor oil

8 ounces coconut oil

22 ounces olive oil

4.41 ounces lye

Red colorant

2-3 ounces peppermint essential oil

Luxurious Vanilla Sugar Scrub Bar

Luxurious vanilla and sugar combine to make a bar that will gently exfoliate.

22.4 ounces lard

9.6 ounces olive oil

12.16 ounces water

4.24 ounces lye

4 vanilla beans, finely chopped (or ground)

1 cup white sugar

2 ounces vanilla fragrance oil

Grandma's Apple Pie Soap

This soap uses the traditional soap ingredient of lard and other ingredients that are easily found at the grocery store to make a soft and cleansing bar that smells just like apple pie.

9.6 ounces Crisco

9.6 ounces olive oil

6.4 ounces lard

6.4 ounces coconut oil

12.16 ounces water

4.463 ounces lye

1/8 cup brown sugar

1 ounce apple pie fragrance oil

¼ cup colloidal oatmeal

2-Pound Hot Process Soap Recipes

For readers who may not want to make as much as 5-pound batches, the following recipes are about 2 pounds each. These are perfect for a 10-inch loaf mold, making about 7-8 4-ounce bars. For hot process soaps, recipes have the same parameters as the others included in this book.

Where's the Beef? Tallow Soap

Like lard, tallow is an animal-based fat used in soap making. It contributes to the hardness of the soap, is conditioning, and has a nice creamy lather. You can choose to leave this soap unscented for a natural smell, or use a fragrance oil of your choice. I like a fall scent like spiced pumpkin or apple cider.

6.7 ounces canola oil

5.3 ounces coconut oil

12 ounces beef tallow

3.34 ounces lye

7.9 ounces water

2 ounces fragrance oil of your choice

Tangerine Shea Butter Soap

The vitamin and mineral content of Shea butter makes it great for dry or sensitive skin. The hot process method is ideal for stabilizing the bright, refreshing tangerine fragrance, ensuring that your scent doesn't fade over time.

5.5 ounces coconut oil

6.6 ounces olive oil

5.5 ounces palm oil

1.7 ounces shea butter

2.6 ounces sweet almond oil

7.2 ounces distilled water

3.09 ounces lye

1.4 ounces tangerine essential oil

3 tsp. dried grated orange peel

Mix in the dried orange peel in the "Personalize" stage.

Charcoal and Clay Facial Bar

This facial soap is great for acne-prone skin of all ages. It gently conditions and cleanses as well as exfoliates with the antibacterial properties of activated charcoal and bentonite clay. The eucalyptus and spearmint essential oil blend gives it a refreshing scent.

2 ounces castor oil

9 ounces coconut oil

9 ounces olive oil

2.9 ounces lye

8 ounces distilled water

1.5 ounces eucalyptus and spearmint essential fragrance oil blend

1 tablespoon activated charcoal powder

1 tablespoon bentonite clay powder

Add the charcoal and clay to your fats before mixing with the lye solution, using the stick blender to incorporate.

Castile Buttermilk Baby Soap

This gentle castile soap is great for sensitive baby's skin, and since it uses the hot process method it cures in half the time. The herbal infused oil imparts a light chamomile scent; if you would like a stronger scent add the chamomile essential oil.

30 ounces olive oil- after infusion, you will use 20.9 ounces for your soap

1.1 ounces castor oil

7.3 ounces buttermilk

2.7 ounces lye

1.5 ounces Dried Chamomile flowers

1.3 ounces chamomile essential oil, optional

To make infused olive oil: On the stovetop, place the dried chamomile flowers and olive oil in a double boiler. Cover and simmer on low for 30 minutes. Let oil cool to room temperature. Since some oil will be absorbed by the botanicals, this recipe allows for extra. Only use 20.9 ounces when making your soap.

Headache Relief Essential Oil Bar

This blend of calming and stimulating essential oils is perfect for an aching head. Take a warm shower with this bar and feel the tension slip away.

6.9 ounces coconut oil

6.9 ounces olive oil

6.9 ounce palm oil

2.3 ounces wheat germ oil

3.3 ounces lye

7.6 ounces distilled water

.4 ounces peppermint essential oil

.2 ounces lavender essential oil

.2 ounces eucalyptus essential oil

.1 ounces rosemary essential oil

Spice Up Your Soap With Fragrances, Colors, and Essential Oils, and More

Here are some quick tips to help you add some zing to your soaps! This information will come in handy if you start to create your own soap recipes (I highly encourage you to do that!). Just follow the instructions from either the cold process or hot process methods, and then add in any of the below additives at the appropriate step!

Fragrance

Fragrance oils are very delicate. For that reason, many do not maintain their integrity during the cold process. Fragrance oils react differently depending on the recipe, so you'll have to experiment a bit when not following a recipe.

Color

Adding color to soap can be tricky. There are a few different types of colorants. The dry colorants include mica (which adds a light sparkle and great color) and pigment (either ultramarines or oxides). 1 teaspoon of mica or pigment colorant per pound of base oil will produce a dark and bold shade. For a pastel, use 1/8 to ¼ of a teaspoon per pound of oils. For best results, mix your color with a small amount of oil or glycerin and blend all the lumps out.

Another form of color is a food dye, which comes in either liquid or powdered form. The amount to use per pound really depends on the type of dye you have bought, so experimentation is good. Start small and work your way up to achieve the color you want.

Sometimes, ingredients in your recipe can actually change the color of your soap, so you might have to adjust. For example, olive oil tends to give soap a greenish color. Fragrance oils can also change the color of soaps, though this is more rare.

Essential Oil

Essential oils add scent and health benefits to your soap. Prices vary from oil to oil, but there is a huge variety out there for you to discover.

Here's a list of some common essential oils listed by health benefits they are said to have. Many oils have incredible benefits, so I encourage you to do your own research.

Acne: Chamomile, Lavender, Lemon, Cedarwood, Clove bud, Grapefruit, Peppermint, Rosemary

Anti-Septic/Anti-bacterial: Basil, Black Pepper, Cedarwood, Clove Bud, Eucalyptus, Ginger, Grapefruit, Orange, Rosemary

Deodorizing: Bergamot, Clary Sage, Lavender, Lemongrass, Pine, Rosewood

Dry Skin: Chamomile, Jasmine, Sandalwood

Insomnia-Lemon Balm, Lavender, Chamomile, Sandalwood, Thyme

Add 3%-5% scent to cold process soaps per pound of base oils. Some essential oils (like anise, cinnamon, clove, or mint) are much stronger than others (like lavender, grapefruit, or chamomile), so keep this in mind when adding your essential oils. Try adding fixatives (like benzoin powder, orris root powder, or different clays) to make your scents last longer.

Other Additives

Herbs, spices, and food items, such as lavender and oatmeal, can lend your soaps great visual appeal and textural qualities.

Minerals such as clays and salts can add color and texture. Bentonite clay, for example, provides a lot of slip and is great for shaving soaps. Use up to one tablespoon per pound of oils. Bentonite can also draw out oils or help fix a scent.

Preservatives

Grapefruit seed extract, rosemary extract, and vitamin E oil can all act as natural preservatives for your home made soap. If you don't want to use preservatives, use the freshest ingredients you can and store your soaps carefully. Keep the superfat level to around 5-10%.

Packaging Your Soap for Gifts or Selling

You can place your homemade soap bars loosely in a cardboard box or plastic container once they have cured completely. Homemade soap does need air circulation to avoid a weepy or rancid soap bar. Adding preservatives to your soap can extend their longevity and add additional beneficial qualities. Assuming proper storage, your homemade soaps should last from half a year to a year. If you plan to give individual soaps out as gifts (or just like to store them individually), wrap them in cotton muslin bags for long-term storage or wrap them in pretty paper if you know they'll be used immediately or if you're selling them.

A cool, dry location will help preserve the soap. Try to keep once scent or scent family per box, as it's likely the scents would muddle together if you put them all in the same box. You don't want your citrus soaps to smell like peppermint! Fragrance oils tend to hold their scent for a year or more, while essential oils tend to degrade a bit faster and last from a few months to half a year. Citrus smells do tend to break down faster, while stronger smells like peppermint last longer.

Conclusion

Thank you so much for reading my book. I hope you feel encouraged to undertake your own soap-making journey after this introduction to making your own soap. Soap can certainly be intimidating, but once you get the hang of it, you'll be making soap for (or with!) all your friends and family. As long as you take the right precautions, you'll find soap making to be an easy and rewarding experience. Soon you'll be ready to experiment with soaps that are more complex!

Book 3:

Homemade Shampoo:

Over 25 Revitalizing, Natural Shampoo Recipes to Give You Healthy, Beautiful Hair

Karen Wells

Table of Contents

Introduction

Hair care may seem like a trivial thing in life to some people, but others know it is actually a very important part of your body's health. Just like your skin, your hair needs to be pampered and cared for to ensure it stays healthy and keeps turning heads wherever you go. It's about much more than just getting that clean feeling after washing your hair... it's about being conscious of your body's overall health and natural beauty.

This starts with the right type of shampoo, which is why it is a shame that most people don't know what is going on inside that bottle. They don't know what it's made of, what chemicals it contains and what damage it might ultimately do in the long run as they lather it into their hair day after day. Making your own shampoo, on the other hand, takes the guesswork out of the process as you can take control of the ingredients that you are putting on your body.

Making your own shampoo will not only allow you to feel guilt free about what you are putting into your hair, you will be able to use it for your children or pets when they take baths and do so with a clean conscience. This is something you can do that is not only good for you and those you love, but something that is good for the environment as well.

Inside you will learn the secrets commercial shampoo manufacturers don't want you to hear and before you know it you will be making some of the smoothest, most loved shampoos you've ever used! Finding ingredients is easier than you may think and with a bit of hunting and a little luck you will be able to create amazing products for a fraction of the cost of fancy store bought shampoos. Who knows, you may even end up with enough left over to sell to others who want the benefits of all-natural shampoo without going through the hassle of making it themselves!

You have already taken the step to a healthier, more beautiful you, now it is time to continue your journey and learn how to make your own shampoo with all natural ingredients that you will be sure to love. It's easier than you might think and in no time you will have healthier, cleaner and more beautiful hair than you ever thought possible.

Chapter 1: Kick Your Store Bought Shampoo to the Curb

Commercial shampoo is a big problem for many people out there: they want clean hair, and yet are afraid or otherwise unwilling to accept the plethora of chemicals that traditional shampoos insist on including in their ingredients list. This can be a problem as these chemicals cause harmful side effects when your body soaks them up, which can lead to a wide variety of unfortunate health concerns. While the results might not come on right away, they can come back later on and cause more serious issues, including cancer.

In many states, there has to be a disclaimer listing any active ingredients that have been shown to cause cancer, but not in every state or for every chemical. This, in turn, can make any trip to buy new hair care products filled with way more anxiety than it has to be.

Here are the most common and most harmful chemicals that are found in shampoos in the industry:
- Sodium Lauryl/Laureth Sulfate (SLS/SLES)
- Dioxane
- Diethanolamine or DEA
- Propylene Glycol
- Parabens

These chemicals have been talked about in many health journals and some of the chemicals are banned from certain countries because of the negative effects that they have on people that try to use them. When it comes to using them for yourself, and your loved ones; do you really want to take the chance of you or they obtaining cancer because someone is rubbing those harmful chemicals into their pores, their scalp, maybe even their eyes, nose or ears.

What's worse, these chemicals are generally just fillers that clean relatively well, smell good and cost a fraction of what natural alternatives would cost in the long run. This, of course, causes companies to use the cheaper method and then charge more for the shampoo. This is what you're buying, and the companies know it but they do not have to disclose that any of the chemicals can harm you, they just have to give you the ingredients list and allow you to do the work if you want. Most people do not want to do the research so they leave it as it is and continue to use it anyway, even with the chemicals in them. This is a convenient way to wash your hair and not have to worry about the effects that might come into play later on down the road.

Many people do not think of the long term and as a result continue to use commercial shampoos as well as soaps, cleaning products, makeup and other products that hold these chemicals in them. Oh yes, do not be deceived into thinking that shampoo is the only product on the market that has these types of chemicals in it. Health products, hygiene products and more all have these chemicals in them and you should be aware of them before you use or purchase the products.

On the contrary, if you want to try your hardest to stay away from these products as time moves forward, consider all of the natural items that you can make for yourself that work just as well, if not better, than the products that you would otherwise purchase at the store.

When you're able to rid yourself of these chemicals, you're able to feel much more confident about the products that you use to get clean with; this comes with knowing what products are in the shampoos you're using to clean your hair. You want something that is going to get the job done, with additional benefits and so much more. Nothing could be better than knowing that you have the perfect shampoo for your needs, which contains nothing but the bare essentials to keep your hair as healthy and beautiful as possible.

One of the most recommended ways to know that you're cleaning, really cleaning your hair, or even your entire body is by making your own shampoo and soaps and cleaning yourself with them. You will know what is in them since you mixed the ingredients on your own. You will know what you're able to get out of them when you clean yourself. You also know that harmful chemicals are not within them.

You can also make your own soap to put your mind at ease. The following chapters will explain the basics of how you can go about doing that with some easy to follow directions and great smelling recipes. You no longer have to spend thousands of dollars in department stores searching for the perfect soaps and shampoos when you know in your heart that none really exist.

The remaining chapters will provide you with the right recipes to get you clean while also making sure you and your loved ones remain as free from chemicals that might harm you in the process as possible. If you want to feel like you're doing something meaningful while still striving to be more natural with the products you use to clean yourself the recipes listed within will help you feel that way, now and for the rest of your life.

It is important to understand that the process of making shampoo on your own is a marathon, not a sprint; slow and steady wins the race. The recipes provided below will set you on the path to a more natural, and ultimately healthier you, but they are not the end of the journey. Use what you have learned within to go out and continue your quest for higher quality soaps and shampoos... your hair awaits you!

Chapter 2: The Wondrous Benefits of Using Homemade Shampoo

Using natural shampoo not only gives you the confidence to say that you know where your ingredients come from; it gives you the ability to have that all over clean feeling without the anxiety of health conditions from chemicals often found in store purchased bottles of shampoo.

What's more, you can use this opportunity to create a signature scent by choosing the perfect scent for your shampoo, as well as the ingredients to ensure the right texture and feel. You can also always mix up the ingredients list so that you're able to find a mixture that works with your type of hair. This is a big consideration to make since everyone wants a shampoo that brings out the natural shine, the curls or the other specifics of their hair. You're able to do this with the right recipe because you have taken matters into your own hands and decided to make your own.

You no longer worry about spending vast sums on hygiene products since you can make your own. You can wash and shampoo and ensure that you get the benefits that you would normally get from store purchased products but without the price or the chemicals that come with them something no one wants when trying to get and stay clean.

Natural shampoo is also something that is high in market demand. Many people will want to try out the shampoo that you make once you let them know more about how you're making it. You will let them know that you're not using harmful chemicals, that the shampoo can be made for specific hair types, and how it is able to condition and smooth without having to purchase extra conditioner in the process.

Natural shampoo is something that can be made right from the comfort of your home. You're able to use it with each and every bath or shower and you can feel good about using it, as well.

Chapter 3: Common Homemade Shampoo Questions Answered

Many people ask this question right off the bat. They want to know that what they are doing is not a waste and that they can feel good about what they are going to spend their time making. If this sounds like you, just know, this shampoo is one of the best things that you can ever do in terms of giving yourself, and your hair a new outlook on life.

Here are some common questions that people ask before they consider starting to make their own shampoo from home.

Can homemade shampoo really clean my hair just as well as store purchased shampoo?

Homemade shampoo is able to clean your hair just as well, if not better than store purchased shampoo. You're able to use soap in the recipe, and an oil that will give the shampoo fragrance that is needed to make your hair smell great after it has been washed. Once you try out the homemade shampoo, you will wonder why you have not washed your hair with it previously. You simply choose the ingredients that you want to use, and go from there.

Will homemade shampoos work for my hair type?

There are so many recipes out there that you can use. Each recipe is for general hair so that anyone is able to use them - great for guests that come to your home or recipes that are specifically made for a hair type. You can look for these types of recipes for yourself, depending on the hair type that you have. You can also make shampoos based on whether you have dry, damaged hair and so on. Just like at the store, you can make a shampoo that is the perfect fit to help your hair.

Are homemade shampoos safe to use on colored/dyed hair?

Homemade shampoos are safe to use on all types of hair and hair types, even hair that has been dyed recently. All-purpose shampoos provide this cleaning solution, but you can also add moisturizing additions, smoothing essentials and the best smells. Each recipe will not wear down the color in your hair, there are no chemicals that will react with the dye and you can get the all over clean that you're looking for.

If you're convinced, then perhaps it might be something you can actually try out for yourself. A natural shampoo that you can make provides you with the all over clean that you're in need of and can open your eyes to a whole new world filled with chemical free, all natural cleaners for your body and your home. Stay safe out there and make sure to get started with the right ingredients that do not hold the types of harmful chemical products that will ultimately cause problems in the future.

While it's true talk is cheap, the results you will get when using a natural shampoo speak for themselves. Do yourself a favor and mix up a small batch, just to try; the difference you will see when it comes to cleanliness, volume, shine and smell will be all the proof you'll need.

Ready to get started?

Chapter 4: Basic Ingredient Overview

Typically, the most initially difficult and time consuming part of the process is determining the right ingredients for you, as well as, your hair. By collecting the necessary ingredients and reading through the list of what you need to do, you can prepare yourself for the process and head out without forgetting anything to make your shampoo. Here are some of the basics that you will need to throw together to create the shampoos that you would like to have. Keep in mind, though, many recipes might call for an additional item that is not on this list. If you're going to be putting together a specific recipe, then it is best to read through that to find out if there is a specific recipe not named here. Remember, forewarned is forearmed.

All of these ingredients are not too hard to find if you know where to look, and, luckily, the list includes that sort of information as well. Remember, all the ingredients should be 100 percent natural without any chemicals added into them to make your shampoo do the job it is supposed to do.

Common Ingredients

Coconut Milk: This is found in grocery stores, health food stores and can be made at home naturally with canned coconut, water and some heat. Coconut is considered a hair superfood thanks to its substantial protein content and a high number of fats. In addition, it produces an anti-microbial, fungal and bacterial oil which adds to the hairs natural silkiness.

Specifically, coconut milk is known to provide a superior form of conditioning, reduce the odds of hair turning gray, naturally cause hair to form looser curls, add to hairs supple nature, improve hair growth, reduce breakage and shredding and improve scalp health. It is also known to combat several more serious scalp issues including dermatitis.

Liquid Castile Soap: This can be found in farmer's markets, health food stores and even online. It is an all-natural soap made from vegetable oil. Originally castile soap was made purely out of olive oil, but today it is made from a wide variety of tallow-free ingredients including a vast array of essential oils to provide a substantial variety.

When choosing a castile soap for the making shampoos, an unscented version is typically best as it can be used with any recipe without clashing without additional scents. A good castile soap choice is one that is made from jojoba oil, hemp oil, coconut oil and water. Due to the wide variety of castile soaps on the market, it is important to carefully consider the ingredients in the one you choose to prevent allergic reactions.

Essential Oils: These can be purchased at a health food store, at some craft stores and even at discounted prices throughout the Internet. You choose the scents you would like your shampoo to have, and you can mix and match to make new scents. Essential oils are one of the oldest known cosmetic products and with good reason; the correct essential oil or mix of essential oils can add a dash of emotionally and spiritually uplifting aromas to any natural shampoo.

Common essential oils include allspice berry, a sweet and spicy aroma that pairs well with cinnamon, ginger and orange. Chamomile is also a natural choice, this mild, sweet fruity aroma has perfume undertones and will last throughout the day

Baking Soda: This is a common ingredient that can be found throughout grocery stores in many different sizes inexpensively. This extremely common cleaner works both to clean the hair and leave it softer than before. This is because of how it reacts when it encounters a low pH. When wet, hair typically has a pH of around 5 which is low enough for it to be considered acidic. The baking soda itself has a pH of around 9 which means it evens out the pH to around a 7, or balanced state. This, in turn, allows the hair to more easily absorb the right amount of water when washed, not too much and not too little for the perfect results every time.

Olive Oil or Other Vegetable Oils: Commonly found in grocery stores among the cooking supplies, when used in a shampoo or conditioner, olive oil and other, similar oils are known to improve the health, strength, shine and overall look of your hair. Oil is a good choice for a natural hair boost because of the way the oil interacts with the hair. It coats each strand individually, working at a molecular level to making it naturally more vibrant than it was before.

Olive oil and other oils are a great choice when it comes to lowering dandruff frequency, stopping the creation of new split ends and repairing existing split end damage. It is also high in vitamin A and vitamin E and scientific research shows that consistent use can restore nutrients to nutrient-deficient hair.

Pure Aloe Vera: This can be found mostly online, but health food stores sometimes carry it since it is also good for many other medical uses as well. When used as a shampoo, pure aloe vera makes a great conditioning agent while at the same time actually repairing any dead skin cells that might be resting on the scalp which means it reduces itching and dandruff. What's more, it helps the hair naturally appear shiner and smoother.

Some tests also show that it improves hair growth when used over a prolonged period of time. When it comes to existing hair, pure aloe vera will also keep it in one place by helping it remain resistant to breaking and improving its elasticity.

Water: This is generally used either warm or room temperature and should be distilled. This can be purchased in bottles this way or you can boil the water to make it distilled and cleaned. While it can sound like an unnecessary hassle to worry about buying or making distilled water prior to making your own shampoo at home, it is important to not underestimate the impurities in tap water. Many of the minerals in tap water are rough on hair, and adding more from the source responsible for cleaning it is only making matters worse.

Just look at the nutrient buildup on most showerheads to determine how pure your water actually is. The goal of all natural shampoos is to give your hair access to the best form of nutrients possible, go the extra mile and use the best water you can.

Honey: Pure, all natural honey can be purchased from farmer's markets and local stands where they raise and harvest bees and honey. Pure honey is what is known as an emollient which means it will naturally help to make your hair softer and healthier. It even helps to stimulate hair growth when used regularly! It does this by ensuring individual hair follicles are as healthy as possible. Studies show that honey can even reactivate some hair follicles that are otherwise dormant.

Honey is also a humectant which means it helps your scalp retain as much moisture as possible which can prevent things like infections or psoriasis which also reduces hair loss.

Stinging Nettle: This extract can be found at most pharmacies as well as online. Despite the name, nettles have been known to improve the health and vitality of hair as well as providing conditioning effects and even stimulating dormant hair growth. In fact, a well-known hair loss remedy is literally nothing more than boiled nettle plant, vinegar and water mixed together and preserved through the use of cologne!

Nettles are also known to mitigate a major cause of hair loss, hormones that are out of balance. They are also high in silica which promotes overall hair health by improving the strength of individual strands which in turn translates to fewer split ends overall.

Lemon: The common lemon is beneficial to hair in numerous ways. When it comes to adding lemon juice to your shampoo, fresh is always better as lemon juice typically contains additives. Lemon juice is a greater choice for a shampoo additive because hair naturally holds on to toxins that leave it discolored and damaged; damage that the acidity lemons naturally fights off.

Lemon will also remove any built up oil deposits while leaving your natural hair oils intact. Even if you don't plan on regularly using it in your shampoos, a good lemon soak now and then is always a healthy choice as it will help to remove excessive buildup that store bought shampoos and conditioners leave behind.

Cucumber: When it comes to using fruits and vegetables in

your shampoo, it is important to always choose organic alternatives to avoiding provide chemicals an avenue reaching your hair and scalp despite your best efforts. Cucumbers are a great choice when it comes to finding a natural way to make your hair fuller and healthier at the same time and helping it to look as smooth and shiny as possible. It contains high amounts of sulphur sodium, calcium, phosphorus, potassium, silicon and manganese, all of which combine to provide a great treatment for nutrient deprived hair. It is also a great natural choice for those looking to mitigate hair loss concerns.

Cornstarch: Yet another common food preparation item on the list, cornstarch is definitely qualified to move from the kitchen to the cosmetics cabinet. Cornstarch's starchy nature makes it ideal for removing stray dirt and oil for hair when in a hurry. It is also known to provide extra strength to individual hair follicles while improving collagen production, leading to smoother, fuller hair. It can also mitigate dryness concerns and increase the hair's antioxidant levels which in turn reduces the presence of free radicals. Vitamin K, present in high amounts in corn starch, is also known to absorb excess calcium, which can ultimately lead to a decreased risk of hair loss when used regularly.

Apple Cider Vinegar: This common bone broth additive is also great when it comes to improving the pH of your hair leaving it smooth and strong. In addition, it is known for sealing small cracks in hair follicles which leaves them soft. This goes a long way towards helping it prevent split ends and repair those already in place. Its acidic nature also makes it a great choice for those with dry, itchy scalps as it will break through any natural or artificial buildup on the scalp and leave it fresh and healthy afterwards. For those dealing with hair that tangles easily, apple cider vinegar is also a natural choice for its detangling agents.

Tea Tree Oil: Available at most grocery stores and pharmacies, tea tree oil is known to help with a wide variety of hair related problems including stimulating hair growth. It is also great for soothing irritated scalps, fixing the issues that cause dandruff and psoriasis and even combat head lice.

Tea tree oil works primarily by unblocking hair follicles while boosting their general immune system thanks to a host of antiviral, antiseptic, antibacterial and antifungal qualities. In addition, the natural qualities of the oil naturally helps the hair to lock in moisture and stay strong for as long as possible. It is also a great additive for baby shampoo as it is known to treat the condition known as cradle cap.

Cognac: Available wherever liquor is sold, this classic liquor will surprise you with how beneficial to your hair it can actually be. It is great when looking to remove unwanted buildup from your scalp while helping to mitigate dandruff concerns as well as itchy scalp. The alcohol will leave your hair looking extremely luscious, shiny and clean. It is also known to help prevent hair loss thanks to its ability to remove toxins and clear follicles to promote hair growth. It should be used in moderation however as too much alcohol in your hair can deplete it of natural oils leaving it dry and limp.

Egg: Another immigrant from the refrigerator, eggs are rich in protein, something your hair will especially love. Extra protein means each individual hair follicle will remain strong in the face of adversity, sealing split ends and preventing new ones from forming in the process.

Protein is also known to leave hair especially shiny and

smooth, an extra boon for those whose hair is typically lifeless and limp. Eggs are also great for creating hair that looks fuller while also acting as a conditioner, locking in excess moisturizer for hair in need of extra moisture. They are also great for those looking for a natural way to detangle especially curly hair.

Avocado: Another in a long line of vegetables as beneficial when applied externally as when eaten. Avocados are a great choice for adding to your personal homemade shampoo as they are especially good at locking moisture into hair, even when faced with intense heat treatment. Avocado oil is also one of few oils strong enough to actually penetrate hair cuticles completely providing results few other ingredients can match.

Avocados are also extremely high in B6, vitamin E, vitamin D and vitamin A as well as iron, copper, folic acid, magnesium, amino acids and proteins, all things that your hair requires in order to look its best. Fresh avocado and avocado oil are equally valid options when it comes to shampoo ingredients.

Rosemary: Not just a common seasoning, rosemary offers a surprising number of benefits when used regularly as part of an all-natural shampoo. When added it large amounts to shampoos it is known to naturally darken the color of the hair while at the same time reducing hair fall and influencing new hair growth.

The ursolic acid found in rosemary is enough to improve blood circulation in the scalp which in turn provide the hair follicles with more of the nutrients and oxygen they need to look and feel their best. It is also a great choice for those looking to prolong going gray as it decreases the chance of new hairs coming in gray.

Once you've gathered these primary ingredients, it is time to ensure that you're ready to go through the steps that are needed to make the shampoo. You want to mix them together, create a soft and luxurious feeling shampoo that you can use in the bath or shower, on yourself and those you love.

Some of the recipes that you will come across use most of these products together, while some only use a few. This is why it is advised that you read the recipes you want to use prior to going out and choosing the ingredients.

If you think of an ingredient that you have heard works great but is not on our list, then feel free to add it. However, this list is a list of ingredients that are chemical free and natural for you to use in the shampoo that you're going to be cleaning your hair with. We cannot guarantee that the ingredient you choose to use is also a natural choice that you can place in the shampoo, so keep this in mind when choosing your choice of ingredients to put in your shampoo.

The goal is to use only the best natural ingredients out there and the only way to do this is by recommending a list that many people found to be useful, while also ensuring that the chemical makeup of the ingredients are natural ones without harmful fillers or other additives that can cause cancer or other ailments when they are used for an extended period of time.

Following easy recipes to make your own shampoo can be done to ensure that you wash your hair in style to make it smell good and look great.

Chapter 5: About the Recipes in This Book

Here are nearly 30 different shampoo recipes that are all perfect for different situations depending on the hair issues you are working to mitigate. Don't forget, the recipes listed below are great, but they should only be considered a template, use what's here but make your own changes to find the perfect shampoo for you and your family. Keep in mind, that the essential oils can be changed to accommodate the scent you would like whether it is a lot or a little.

This is your shampoo and you can have it anyway that you'd like to use it. Feel free to experiment with more or less oil, more coconut milk or your choice of soap mixtures. Have fun with the process and know that this is something that doesn't take a lot of patience or even skill to make. You can make what you like easily and use it to your advantage.

The following recipes will start with explaining the best usage scenario for each recipe, provide you with the necessary ingredients and then lists any preparation tips that may be required. None of these recipes require more than 10 minutes of preparation and they can all be made right from the comfort of your own home.

Storing your shampoo

Storing your shampoos is an important part of the process. What's more, every shampoo is different because of the ingredients which it contains. A general guideline for the shelf life of shampoo is to write down the day that it was mixed together and do not use it a month after that date. Make sure you are aware of the shelf-life of anything you add to your shampoo or one morning you might be in for a nasty surprise!

While freezing will sometimes help with consistency, as a general rule, no all natural shampoo has any specific refrigeration requirements. They can be stored in a cool place, wet place or even a hot place such as the shower. When it comes time to use, you can just grab it off the shelf the same as any store bought version. It really is that easy and it provides you with an all over clean that doesn't require much storage or a lot of work to achieve.

The bottles that you can store the shampoo in can matter, as well depending on the ingredients. Regardless, you will want to check to see if the bottles are BPA free as otherwise they could leach into your shampoo and ruin all of your hard work when it comes to cleaning yourself naturally. Glass bottles are also a solution, just be careful with them in the shower! The shampoo can slip right out of the bottle and you're able to wash and reuse them as many times as necessary. These bottles can be purchased either online or at a local craft store.

Check for local coupons and deals to get a deal on these bottles. You can go with some of the larger ones or smaller ones. Department stores might have travel bottles that you can fill and use while on the go or to just place in the shower and use. Many people choose to reuse the bottles that hold the shampoo in them. You would just have to clean out a few of them and then fill them with the shampoo that you make right from home. The type of bottle you use is up to you and your specific wants and needs.

Consider decorating the outside of the shampoo bottles with a design that you like. Use specific labels on the outside and write down what the shampoo is, the scents and when it was put together. This can provide you with a way to keep things organized and know what they are and what they are used for and can give others using the shower a heads up, as well.

Have fun...

Simple Suds Shampoo

This is just about the cheapest, quickest and easiest to make shampoo imaginable. What's even better, you are practically guaranteed to have all of the required ingredients in your home right now.

Preparation Time: Less than 60 seconds.

Ingredients:
1 tablespoon of baking soda
1 cup of warm water

- **Directions:**
  Place the baking soda in a bottle of warm water and shake thoroughly.
- Shake before each use to remove clumps.

No More Tangles Nourishing Shampoo

Smells great smooths out the most tangled hair and is gentle enough to use on children's scalps.

Preparation Time: 5 minutes

Ingredients:
1/4 cup of coconut milk
1/3 cup of the liquid Castile soap
20 drops of your own favorite essential oils
Add a teaspoon of olive or almond oil for dry hair types (optional)

Directions:
- Combine all of the ingredients in a shampoo bottle of your choice. You can clean out an old one or purchase squeeze bottles from most pharmacies.
- Shake the bottle well each time prior to use to ensure ingredients remain well combined.
- Each batch should last up to a month and can be stored in the shower
- Most people will only need a teaspoon per use

Voluptuous Volume Shampoo

A great way to nourish the hair and make it appear thicker than it is.

Preparation Time: 5 minutes

Ingredients:
1/4 cup of distilled water
1/4 cup of liquid Castile soap
1/2 teaspoon of jojoba, olive, or grape seed oil

Directions:
- Mix the ingredients together until smooth and pour into a bottle.
- Each batch should last up to a month and can be stored in the shower
- Most people will only need a teaspoon per use

Oily Remedy Shampoo

For unmanageable, oily hair that needs to be tamed.

Preparation Time: 5 minutes, freeze for a few hours.

Ingredients:
1 can of coconut milk
1 3/4 cups of pure aloe vera gel
Essential oils of your choice

Directions:
- Mix the ingredients together fully using a whisk
- Pour the mixture into ice cube trays and put in the fridge for a few hours.
- When they are tougher, put them in a bag or container in the freezer.
- Take one or two out and put it in a container on the counter an hour or so before use.

Silky Smooth Shampoo with Essentials

Provides an all over smooth, yet nourishing appeal using honey and other natural oils.

Preparation Time: 5 minutes

Ingredients:
1/2 cup of liquid castile soap
1/4 cup of coconut milk
1/4 cup of honey
2 tablespoons of coconut oil
1 tablespoon of vitamin E oil
50 drops of essential oils of your choice

Directions:

- Shake the bottle well each time prior to use to ensure ingredients remain well combined.
- Each batch should last up to a month and can be stored in the shower
- Most people will only need a teaspoon per use

Castile Olde Style Shampoo

Quick, old-style shampoo with your choice of scent using essential oils.

Preparation Time: 3 minutes

Ingredients:
1/2 cup of liquid castile soap
1 cup of warm water
20 drop of essential oil of your choice (optional)

Directions:
- Shake both of the ingredients together thoroughly to dissolve the soap with the water.

Destroy That Dandruff Shampoo

Rid your hair from dandruff that can flake, look bad and cause you to itch.

Preparation Time: 5 minutes

Ingredients:
1/2 cup of liquid castile soap
1 cup of warm water
10 equal drops of cedar wood, clary sage, lemon, rosemary and tea tree oil

Directions:
- Shake the bottle well each time prior to use to ensure ingredients remain well combined.
- Each batch should last up to a month and can be stored in the shower
- Most people will only need a teaspoon per use

Deliver Us from Dryness Shampoo

Having dry hair is never a good thing, give it a kiss of moisture using this shampoo recipe.

Preparation Time: 5 minutes

Ingredients:
1/2 cup of liquid castile soap
1 cup of warm water
10 equal drops of cedar wood, clary sage, lemon, rosemary and tea tree oil

Directions:
- Shake the bottle well each time prior to use to ensure ingredients remain well combined.
- Each batch should last up to a month and can be stored in the shower
- Most people will only need a teaspoon per use

Tangled Hair Shampoo

When your hair is in knots, you need a shampoo and conditioning agent that is going to smooth it out.

Preparation Time: 5 minutes

Ingredients:
1/2 cup of liquid castile soap
1 cup of warm water
10 equal drops of chamomile, grapefruit, passionflower, marigold and sweet clover
Add a small dab of aloe vera
Teaspoon of olive oil or coconut oil for shine

Directions:
- Shake the bottle well each time prior to use to ensure ingredients remain well combined.
- Each batch should last up to a month and can be stored in the shower
- Most people will only need a teaspoon per use

Gentle Lavender Lemongrass Shampoo

Preparation Time: 5 minutes

Ingredients:
1 oz. liquid castile soap
4 oz. filtered water
3 drops lavender essential oil
3 drops orange essential oil
3 drops lemongrass essential oil

Directions:
- Shake the bottle well each time prior to use to ensure ingredients remain well combined.
- Each batch should last up to a month and can be stored in the shower
- Most people will only need a teaspoon per use

Thin to Thick Shampoo

Thin hair is not what most people want, and if that's you then this recipe is something that you don't want to miss – it will help your hair get that fuller appearance you're looking for.

Preparation Time: 5 minutes

Ingredients:
1/2 cup of liquid castile soap
1 cup of warm water
20 equal drops of clary sage and cedar wood

Directions:
- Shake the bottle well each time prior to use to ensure ingredients remain well combined.
- Each batch should last up to a month and can be stored in the shower
- Most people will only need a teaspoon per use

Neutralizing Shampoo

Some people may just have naturally oily hair, and while this might be okay for a day but leaving it any longer can become noticeable.

Preparation Time: 5 minutes

Ingredients:
1/2 cup of liquid castile soap
1 cup of warm water
10 equal drops of cedar wood, lavender, pine, rosemary

Directions:
- Shake the bottle well each time prior to use to ensure ingredients remain well combined.
- Each batch should last up to a month and can be stored in the shower
- Most people will only need a teaspoon per use
- Smooth over the hair and leave in for two minutes before rinsing.

Moisturizing Shampoo

Dry, dull hair will need a kiss of moisture and with the right ingredients, you can add this to your hair without a problem.

Preparation Time: 5 minutes

Ingredients:
1/2 cup of liquid castile soap
1 cup of warm water
10 equal drops of thyme, cedar wood, ylang-ylang or clary sage
1/3 cup of coconut milk
2 tablespoons of coconut or olive oil

Directions:
- Shake the bottle well each time prior to use to ensure ingredients remain well combined.
- Each batch should last up to a month and can be stored in the shower
- Most people will only need a teaspoon per use
- For a milkier, thicker consistency, consider whisking the ingredients together instead

Shiny Luster Shampoo

Luster, shine and brilliance are what each woman wants for their hair and you can have it with the right mixture of shampoo ingredients.

Preparation Time: 5 minutes

Ingredients:
1/2 cup of liquid castile soap
1 cup of warm water
1 tablespoon of coconut milk
1 tablespoon of pure aloe vera
20 equal drops of sweet basil and Roman chamomile

Directions:
- Shake the bottle well each time prior to use to ensure ingredients remain well combined.
- Each batch should last up to a month and can be stored in the shower
- Most people will only need a teaspoon per use

Waterless Cleansing Shampoo

If you do not want to wash using water, then washing with a dry shampoo can be done. This is perfect for on the go when you have no shower head or sink.

Preparation Time: 5 minutes

Ingredients:
1 tablespoon of salt
1/2 cup of cornmeal
1 teaspoon of baby powder

Directions:
- Mix in a shaker bottle completely before using.
- Shake onto the hair and then brush through to get rid of the oil, dirt and debris.

Raw Honey Shampoo

Beautiful and great smelling hair can be found when you use this shampoo. With nourishing effects and a smooth honey texture, your hair will love what you've done to it.

Preparation Time: 10 minutes

Ingredients:
1 tablespoon of raw honey
3 tablespoons of filtered water
10 drops of essential oils

Directions:
- Sometimes the honey needs a little help to melt and mix with the water. Using hot water can help with the mixing but if you only have cold water available, then put the honey and water together and heat up slightly while stirring until it is fully mixed together.

- Add the essential oils after and shake together.

- Each batch should last up to a month and can be stored in the shower .
- Use a tablespoon or two on the scalp of the hair - no need to reach the ends.

Stinging Nettle Hair Growth Shampoo

While it may sound surprising, applying this stinging nettle based shampoo should allow you to start seeing new hair growth in about a month.

Preparation Time: 5 minutes

Ingredients:
2 tablespoons panthenol solution
25 ml stinging nettle extract
2 vials Vitamin B Complex
50 ml castor oil

Directions:

- Combine all of the ingredients together and mix well, mixing well each time before use.
- Make sure you store the results in a glass jar to prevent herb interaction.
- Use regularly for 4 months for best results.

Cucumber and Lemon Shampoo

This shampoo combines the reinvigorating properties of cucumber with the natural cleaning power of lemon to great result. This shampoo isn't one you'd want to use every day but is great for fighting dandruff.

Preparation Time: 5 minutes

Ingredients:
1 lemon
1 cucumber

Directions:
- Peel both ingredients and add them to a food processor.
- You will know it is finished when the results have become a smooth paste with a runny consistency.
- Be sure to rise your hair well as lemon pulp can be difficult to remove.

Cornstarch Shampoo

Cornstarch makes an effective shampoo either as an alternative to dry shampoos or as an ingredient in an all-natural shampoo that promotes thicker hair. Dry cornstarch shampoo is literally just cornstarch, rub it into your hair and brush it out to remove dirt and oils.

Cornstarch Thickening Shampoo
Preparation Time: 5 minutes

Ingredients:
1 tablespoon baking soda
1 cup of water
Cornstarch as needed

Directions:
- This shampoo is simply a stronger version of the Simple Suds shampoo, mix up the Simple Suds and add cornstarch until it reaches the consistency you require.
- Each batch should last up to a month and can be stored in the shower.
- Most people will only need a teaspoon per use.

All Natural Shampoo and Conditioner

This all natural shampoo variety also conditions as its cleaning, allowing you to be twice as free of chemicals and say twice as much money when compared with store bought brands.

Preparation Time: 5 minutes

Ingredients:
¼ cup water
1 tablespoon tea tree oil
2 tablespoons of apple cider vinegar
1 cup organic liquid castile soap

Directions:
- Add all of the ingredients together in a spray bottle.
- Add 10 drops of an essential oil.
- Each batch should last up to a month and can be stored in the shower

Coconut Milk Shampoo

Coconut shampoo is great for those with drier hair because of its natural conditioning properties.

Preparation Time: 5 minutes

Ingredients:
10 drops of essential oil
1 tablespoon almond oil
1 cup organic liquid castile soap
¼ cup coconut milk

Directions:

- Combine all of the ingredients together and mix well, mixing well each time before use.
- Each batch should last up to a month and can be stored in the shower
- Most people will only need a teaspoon per use

Honey and Cognac Shampoo

While many people have heard of the egg and cognac hair mask, fewer people have gone on to consider using cognac in a traditional shampoo. This is a shame as cognac is great for the scalp and makes an ideal shampoo for normal hair.

Preparation Time: 5 minutes

Ingredients:
1 cup organic liquid castile soap
1 tablespoon honey
1 small glass of cognac

Directions:
- This recipe needs to be prepared prior to each use.
- Mix all of the ingredients together, stir well and add to hair.
- Let sit for 5 minutes prior to rinsing.

Natural Shampoo for Swimmers

This all natural shampoo is ideal for those who plan to spend the summer poolside or at the beach. What's more, you only need to use it once a week to keep your hair looking great all summer.

Preparation Time: 15 minutes

Ingredients:
¼ cup avocado oil
4 oz. castile flakes
¼ gallon of water

Directions:
- Add the water to a large pot and place it on a burner over a high heat to allow it to boil.
- After the water has boiled, add in the flakes and continue stirring until the water cooils.
- Add in the oil, shake well, and shake again prior to each use.
- Each batch should last up to a month and can be stored in the shower.
- Most people will only need a teaspoon per use.

Rosemary Lemon Shampoo

Better than any store-bought shampoos, lemons have the power to really bring out the shine in even the dullest hair.

Preparation Time: 15 minutes

Ingredients:
1/4 cup organic liquid castile soap
½ teaspoon lemon essential oil
2 tablespoons almond oil
2 tablespoons dried rosemary
¼ cup distilled water

Directions:
- Add the water to a large pot and place it on a burner over a high heat to allow it to boil.
- After the water has boiled, add the dried rosemary and and steep until partially cooled.
- Strain the results, combine all of the ingredients together and mix well, mixing well each time before use.
- Each batch should last up to a month and can be stored in the shower.
- Most people will only need a teaspoon per use.

Apple Cider Shampoo

Apple cider vinegar shampoo is an excellent way to get rid of any waxy build up that may appear on the scalp, it also works great for cutting through tough dandruff.

Preparation Time: 5 minutes

Ingredients:
30 ml olive oil
1 teaspoon apple cider vinegar
2 tablespoons lemon juice
1 egg

Directions:
- This recipe needs to be prepared prior to each use.
- Add all of the ingredients to a food processor and mix well

Egg Shampoo

This simple mixture of common household items can lead to surprising results. This moisturizing shampoo is great for all types of hair.

Preparation Time: 5 minutes

Ingredients:
2 teaspoons lemon juice
2 teaspoons olive oil
3 teaspoons of baking soda
2 eggs

Directions:
- This recipe needs to be prepared prior to each use.
- Beat the eggs well before combining all of the ingredients together.
- Use the shampoo to scrub the scalp vigorously before rinsing well.

Conclusion

Now that you've read through the recipes, hopefully, there are at least three or four that you can't wait to try! You can, of course, mix and match the many essential oils that are out there to come up with a truly unique scent of your own. This is something that you can do on your own, experiment with and even speak with other fellow shampoo makers to find out what their thoughts are on making the shampoo without the added chemicals that come with the store purchased versions.

Hopefully, you will have fun making your own shampoo and the effects it will have on your hair compared to the store purchased shampoos that are on the market currently. Make sure to share your recipes with those you know so everyone can get in on the fun.

Homemade, all natural shampoo is something that has been made for years and its popularity is only increasing. Natural shampoo is something that is needed to clean hair, but also to rid your body of those chemicals discussed in chapter 1. It is important to feel comfortable with the shampoo making process, and as such, it is best to start off with a small trial batch, just to be safe.

Thank for making it through to the end of this book, let's hope it was informative and was able to provide you with all of the tools you need. Now it is time for you to get started making the best shampoo that you've ever used. When you can't find one you love in the stores, nothing is stopping you from creating the one that you love to use on your own.

Please, share your questions, comments and love of the book with others that you know and let them know that you can have all natural shampoo without the dangerous chemicals in them. You no longer have to live in fear knowing that you're rubbing those chemicals that could be harming you into your scalp with each and every shower that you take.

I wish you the best on your shampoo making journey and hope that you've learned a lot from what this book has provided!

Book 4:

Homemade Bath Bombs:

The Complete DIY Guide to Making Luxurious, Soothing Bath Bombs

Karen Wells

Table of Contents

Introduction

To begin with I would like to both thank you and congratulate you for downloading this book!

The notion of using essential oils and other soothing elements in one's bath water is a French notion that has been around since the 1930's! With time the 'notion' was soon renamed aromatherapy and by the 1980's it had become common practice, which is how in the late 1980's the rudimentary concept of a bath bomb was created by Mo Constantine, one of the founders of the cosmetics giant Lush. Unfortunately going out and spending oodles of money on high end products isn't in everyone's budget, which of course is why God created DIY's!

This very book contains, in addition to a brief summary on the various health benefits of bath bombs, the entire outline of how one would go about making one, from scratch. The book also includes thirty original recipes, which are tailored to fit in with the needs of each individual reader!

Besides, not only are DIY's great opportunities to test your creative borders they are also light on the wallet, allowing you to indulge in, or give as a gift, things that would normally be out of your reach – Ready to indulge then?

Yes?

Great!

We'll kick off in just a minute but for now, thanks again for downloading this book, I hope you enjoy it!

Chapter 1: The Rejuvinating Benefits of Homemade Bath Bombs

Before we start off on the benefits of 'homemade' bath bombs, let's have a little chat about why we don't just save ourselves the hassle of making these and just, buy them online or something. It sounds like a brilliant idea.

After all with today's day and age long soak in the bath, with that little something extra, is sometimes as close as we can get to actually getting a break especially, if we are college students on a budget or new moms struggling with finances and baby diapers. Unfortunately the fact of the matter is, even a proper soak can be expensive once we have factored in the rising prices for bath-salts, or industry made bath-bombs – with most companies pricing bath bombs at five to six dollars each, it tends to add up to a luxury most of us can't afford.

Right?

Wrong.

This is where DIY's come to play. Not only do homemade bath bombs help us make our own affordable range of luxury items, it also helps us tailor the recipe for the bomb to suit our precise needs!

How?

Well, bath bombs, among other things, are basically a convenient form of aromatherapy. Have you ever wondered why you feel so much better after you light certain scented candles, or why lavender oil is used as a salve for burns or even why a cup of mint tea can instantly make you feel so much better?

It all comes down tot the power of one's olfactory senses - or in short, one's sense of smell. Aromatherapy is a form of holistic healing that is conducted through the use of special essential oils, such as almond, lavender, mint etc. – that is targeted at one's mind and body. Not only are these oils used to give you a physical sense of comfort, but their aromas have a way of helping soothe one's mind as well. By forcing the body to relax, the excess energy instead starts up an innate healing practice within itself, that helps bring back balance to the individual in question.

What's more is, certain essential oils such as bergamot and grapefruit tend to have great moisturizing benefits and can leave you looking years younger after just a few baths!

Now that is real rejuvenation!

And just like that, you get to create your own spa experience - on a budget, without having to shell out hundreds of dollars in yearly bath luxuries!

Chapter 2: All You Need to Know About Making Bath Bombs

As a novice to the art of bath bomb construction it is easy to feel overwhelmed by the many intricacies that are such an inherent part of the process, but for starters all you really need to do is take a minute and breathe!

No, but seriously, this is hardly the end of he world and if you start putting yourself in a panic before we evens tart making bath bombs, then you're basically negating the entire process of creating an object that is supposed to help you de-stress! You are also probably scaring yourself silly – so seriously – just breathe for a minute!

Instead let's be practical and approach this scientifically, we know what a bath bomb is but do we understand how and why it works the way it does?

No?

We'll start there, and then we'll even take a quick detour and help you figure out exactly what you are going to need when you start making them and where you can the materials at the best prices! And if you promise to shake off all the negativity, we'll even give you a peek at some of the secret ingredients that can help you spice up your bath bombs just a bit!

Deal?

Here we go!

What Makes 'Bath Bombs' – 'Bath Bombs'!

Let's talk about magic for a second – we say magic because when your bath bomb hits your bath water and you are covered in that endless fizz, that incredible feeling has got to be magic, right?

Well – only partially – most of it is basic science and that means it can be replicated, right here, right now in the comfort of your home! How amazing is that?

Bath bombs are made up a multitude of basic ingredients that we will talk about later, but the two active ingredients that help create that basic fizz factor are the acidic base and the alkali. It can't just be any alkali though it has to bicarbonate, so that when the combination hits water it can create a chemical reaction that releases carbon dioxide! Or in other words, magic fizz!

Most bath bombs use a weak organic acid, such as citric acid, this is available in the form of a white crystalline powered that is often used as a preservative in most cosmetic products. Cream of Tartar is an easy alternative for citric acid, and just needs to be mixed in at a 2:1 ratio. Some of the other common substitutes include lemon juice or even a sachet of Emergen-C, the fizzy drink, the latter is great if you want to make your bath bombs a child friendly activity, something you could do with your kids or students for instance.

Next up you have the alkali, or to be specific Bicarbonate of Soda, also commonly known as baking soda. The bicarbonate is the one ingredient that cannot be substituted, you see, the organic form of baking soda, derives from Nahcolite, which due to it's bi-carbon formulation is what reacts with the acid and water to basically release carbon dioxide bubbles! The best part is, none of this works until the water is added so you can pack your bath bombs, obviously minus the water and leave them somewhere dry to use whenever you want!

Pretty cool, huh?

Well don't get too excited, that is still just the start, in order for you to make the perfect bath bomb you are going to need a few more ingredients, so why don't you grab yourself a pen and paper while we give you a list of exactly what you are going to need and the best places to find them.

Basic Bath Bomb Supplies – And the Best Deals!

Now that we know all about the science behind Bath-Bombs, we are going to set out a little list of basic supplies so that you can gather everything together before we get to work. To make it easier we'll also tell you where the best deals are so that your little DIY project can be as budget friendly as possible.

(1) Baking Soda

The very first thing on your Bath Bomb ingredients list is – Baking Soda. Now, when it comes to baking soda you can always use the regular stuff you get in the shops, but if you are interested in keeping it purely organic, it's best that you get one that isn't treated by chemicals.

Bob's Red Mill Baking Soda is the best-priced organic Baking Soda available online and is even aluminum free! Just looks it up on Amazon under Cooking and Baking products. If however you don't want to order online, simply go to the nearest Whole Foods or corner grocery and you can compare prices and pick out the one you like best.

(2) Citric Acid/Cream of Tartar

While most bath bomb recipes call for citric acid, we've already explained to you how in some cases citric acid can be replaced with cream of tartar. As ingredients though you now need to focus on where you are going to collect them from.

Citric Acid is a kitchen staple, so odds are you probably already have some in your kitchen, that you use for preserving, flavouring or even cleaning – if not however you are going to want to go with something that is one hundred percent food grade since the product may seep into your skin while you are soaking yourself. We recommend, Milliard 100% Pure Food Grade Citric Acid, also available on Amazon.

Cream of Tartar is similarly also a kitchen staple, however if you don't have any, you can try Badia's Cream of Tartar, which is the number one best seller online, and great bang for your buck if you are going to need it in bulk.

Also as a pro tip, keep in mind that for bulk products it's usually cheapest to buy online, but if you just want to test out the recipe, just get yourself a small box from the supermarket and you can use that.

(3) Water

Well, water hardly needs much explanation, but you are going to need a nice spray bottle for your water so that you don't accidently put in too much. Regular cleaners can be emptied out and used as a water bottle as well if you'd rather cut corners.

These top three round up our basic ingredients, but they are not all that your bath bombs are made of, following as a short list of optional ingredients that you can use to spice up your bath bomb and turn your bath time fun into a real treat of the senses!

(1) Epsom Salts

Magnesium deficits are a growing concern, and one that has an unfortunate tendency to manifest with age. With all the great health benefits magnesium has, starting from fighting off inflammation, improving blood flow and oxygen flow all the way up to fighting off fungi, this is a loss that is keenly if silently felt.

A great way to help counter balance this deficient is to add some Epsom Salt to your bath time fun. Bathing in Epsom Salt allows the magnesium and sulphate to be absorbed into your skin, while simultaneously pulling out harmful toxins.

Ultra Epsom has a great variety of salt grains to choose from, the medical grade, extra fine, (0.0-0.3 mm) is the suggested variety for bath salts fizzies. If you don't want to go for a bulk buy you can buy regular Epsom Salts and then simply grind them finely at home.

(2) Coconut Oil

Coconut oil is another great additive, while not an essential element to the bath bomb, it has so many great benefits, starting from acting as a great moisturizer, to definitive healing powers such as helping prevent or even clear up sunburn, cold sores, eczema and acne.

Once the oil starts soaking into your skin on a regular basis it is even known to help boost metabolism, and help both weight loss and your immune system. Shrinking pores to dandruff, coconut oil literally does it all – which is why coconut oil is such a great addition to your bath bombs.

When you choose what coconut oil to use, it is best to go with something that has been through minimal processing with maximum nutrition. Also if you don't want to add in any additional scents go for one that has a rich aroma – the best option for these particular needs are something that is organic, extra virgin and definitely cold pressed.

Nutiva has a great Organic Coconut oil, and its even hexane free, which makes it my top choice, alternative's Island's Miracle is also great for bulk purchases.

(3) Corn Starch

While corn starch is not a staple for commercial producers and an unnecessary added expenditure for small business's if you are making the bath bombs for yourself or for friends, adding the right amount of corn starch can help the bomb float on water, which is a great visual effect and more importantly works great as a skin softener. It can on occasion aggravate yeast infections though so you may want to avoid them if you are suffering from any.

Once again, we are going to recommend Bob's Red Mill Corn Starch, which is a great price at just about three dollars per twenty-two ounces.

(4) Essential Oils

Essential Oil's a re the very best part of a proper bath bomb, not only do they help you add a zing to you bath bomb, but the right blend and the right oil could even help you help balance your mood or help with your insomnia. As will all products you are recommended to use food grade products since they are the least polluted. Following is a simple chart of uses for Essential Oil so that you can pick and choose which one's you would like to include in your bath bomb.

Depression/Grief - Depression itself is a tough battle to fight as is grief, a good soak is always helpful, so are oils like, Bergamot, Clary Sage, Lemon, Ylang Ylang, Rose, Lavender, Grapefruit, Cypress, Frankincense, and Neroli.

Insecurity/Panic Attacks and Stress Reduction – A few other hard to deal with body and soul battles are insecurity, and stress. Panic attacks generally are induced by stress so the following oils help with all three of these – Cedarwood, Jasmine, Sandalwood, Helicysum, Palo Santo, Patchouli and Chammomile.

Anger Management and Peace and Happiness – Another moment when you absolutely need a soak is when you are pissed off beyond your imagination. And there in that moment all you want is something to calm you down, to help you let go of some of that rage for just a moment, we recommend – Petitgrain, Orange, Neroli, Roman Chamomile, Grapefruit, Sandal wood, and Peppermint.

Also if you want to make a bath bomb for your man, try something non-floral, we recommend – Myrtle, Vanilla, Tobacco, Spruce, Cinnamon, Black Pepper, and Blue Cypress – trust us your man won't know what hit him!

(5) Fragrance

Most bath bomb makers tend to out and out dislike fragrances, mostly because in such close contact the fragrances tend to stick a lot more than they would in a bar of soap or similar DIY projects, but if you want you can try experimenting with left over perfumes or fragrance oils, just make sure you don't go with anything with a cloying scent, no one wants to walk out of bath smelling like chemicals after all.

(6) Coloring

And finally we have coloring – now, while coloring is hardly the most significant part of the process of making bath bombs – it does always add a bit of pop too the product. Now keep in mind the bombs don't look too bad on their own either, they come out with a fresh white linen vibe, but if you want you could consider adding very small amounts of food coloring, (anything else would stain, and no one looks good in green!) or alternatively coloured fruit juices like blueberry or maybe beet juice. This may however affect the life of the bath bomb, so if you are making it for a friend it's probably best to use coloring instead of natural food dyes.

And that sums up all the nifty ingredients you'll be needing for your bath bomb DIY, think of it as you setting up your own mini factory at home! Which is why we recommend that you collect them all, and maybe a few molds (Easter eggs or old plastic balls that can be opened and closed work well) which you could adapt, such as candy molds or Christmas ornament molds, and get them all together before you set up for your own little DIY project!

Chapter 3: The Simple Process for Making Luxurious Bath Bombs

Now that we are about to start the actual process of bath bomb making, we need to do a quick check and make sure we have everything we need. Despite how it sounds bath bombs are generally not a very fussy activity, however in addition to the list of ingredients there is also a short list of must-haves, accompanied of course by a detailed list of instructions that tell us exactly when and how each of our components need to be used in order to properly create and store the bath bomb mixtures.

Step One – Collecting the Supplies and Ingredients

The very first things on our list of mixing essentials are – *measuring cups*! Yes, yes, I know that was obvious, and you probably already knew that but, now we are also going to need to pick up a nice sieve, a spray bottle, tissue paper and molds. You are also going to need a few big bowls, and a dropper for the oil.

Once you've done all that the very first thing, you need to do is make sure that you have everything on hand. Go through your recipe multiple times and check that all of your must haves are at hand – remember having to go look for the water spray half way through the recipe, or realizing you don't have your oils when you start shaping your molds is, trite as it may sound, basically a recipe for disaster.

Step Two – Mixing it all Together

Before you start mixing all your products together it is important that you understand how the composite mixture needs to stand. Your base products are always going to be citric acid and baking soda, now it is imperative that while you can add in a multitude of other elements the 1:1 ratio of citric acid and baking soda is not compromised. If you absolutely must you can substitute some of the citric acid, although this may affect the fizz, just remember to never, ever replace any of the baking soda. The baking soda, is what helps soften the water as well as temper the citric acid, without it the acid has severe irritation possibilities. Just keep that in mind as we talk you through the rest.

Okay? - Great!

Back to basics then – grab your bowl and measure out your baking soda and citric acid in a 1:1 ratio. If you have any other dry ingredients, such as cornstarch that you would like to add, stir them in now. Once that is done, scoop up a tiny amount and put in in a separate bowl, in this separate bowl and add in your coloring and then your essential oils or other liquid ingredients. Some people prefer to mix the liquid elements separately and then add them in to the mixture. While doing so keep in mind you need to mix vigorously, any clumps will ruin the surface of your bath bombs with uneven ridges or cracks. Once you have mixed in all the ingredients, very carefully using only one spray at a time, add water. It is important that you not pour the water and use a water spray so that you may evenly distribute the moisture until your mixture starts to hold together when packed into a ball.

The best way to do this is spray, mix, test and then continuously repeat the process until you have the required consistency. Keep in mind the mixture is not intended to look or feel wet – merely moist enough to hold, they must remain sufficiently dry or else the fizz factor will dissipate. Also don't forget to use gloves!

Step Three – How to Mold and Shape Your Bath Bombs Successfully

Now, once you are all done with our mixing you finally arrive at the final stage of your bath bomb making, well there is still the storing but that's hardly a part of the construction process. Coming back to the point, for your final step you are going to need to get yourself a fixed mold so that the bath bombs can take shape. Generally the bath bombs tend to work better if they are smaller or medium sized, the larger bombs have a tendency to crumble, mostly because your ingredients are packed in together instead of welded together with water.

However, once you have selected a mold, what you need to do is pack it in with the mixture. If you are using a two part mold make sure that the mold is packed in as tightly as you can, stuff it to the gills, press down and just hold it in place until it starts to take shape. Once it has, easily bend the mold to get the bath bombs out, keep I mind that the bath bombs are very fragile so you are not going to want to use hard molds, softer bendable molds with curved surfaces tend to work best. When you are trying to press them out make sure you are just pressing ad not tapping, tapping will make your bath bobs crumble or crack, so remember just press!

Once you've managed to get your bath bombs out, you are going to want to dry them out a bit. It's best to use tissue paper and line a tray or something and then place the newly formed bath bombs on them, spaced out. For better results, pack a bit of tissue in between each of the bath bombs and then cover them with another sheet of tissue paper. Now, leave them out to dry for about a day, use a nice dry place, but avoid direct sunlight since it will crack the bombs or dry them out too much and cause them to break apart entirely.

Step Four– Storing Your Bath Bombs

Now that you've prepared yourself a nice set of bath bombs the only question left is what do you do with them Well there is the obvious – use them but there are other things you can do as well, such as give them away as Christmas gifts, or sell them, all of which will be talked about as soon as we first deal with how to store them.

As you already know it is important that your bath bombs be kept in a dry environment without any direct sunlight. What is also important is ensuring that the products remain airtight for as long as possible. Your best bet is glass jars, also if you do intend on giving these away as gifts glass jars or mason jars can be dressed up to look pretty fancy, although if it is just for personal use you can also try using plastic bags. Even so try not to wait too long before you use your bath bombs they have a more potent effect if they are used quickly and quite frankly sometimes mixing n additional ingredients such as oils, or dried flowers can make the bath bombs go bad quickly.

If you do want to give them away as gifts or sell them you should include these instructions on a little card, explaining how the bath bombs should be used as soon as possible to maximize the fizz and also to store them in dry, cool places without direct sunlight.

So, mixing, molding and storing, just like that you have just made your very first batch of bath bombs! Congratulations!

Chapter 4: 30 Amazing DIY Bath Bomb Recipes

Now that you know how to make your bath bombs, how to store them and what you are going to do with them once you are done making them the only thing left to do is hand you a nice fat Chapter exclusively on bath bomb recipes!

For the sake of diversity we are going to give you a few different types of recipes, some with citric acid, some with cream of tartar, and of course a plethora of essential oils and other components – all you have to do is read through and figure out which one suits your at the moment.

Excited?

Here we go! Also keep in mind, all of the recipes that follow make exactly one bath bomb each, so feel free to alternate the recipe as needed!

Cream of Tartar Bases

1. Spring Blooms

Beautifully infused with Lavender and Mandarin essential oils, this bath bombs will leave you feeling like you are soaking in the very best of spring, with all the flowers and the fruits just bursting back in!

For this recipe you are going to need -

- 2 tablespoons baking soda

- 1/2 tablespoon cream of tartar

- 1 tablespoon of cornstarch

- 1 tablespoon Epsom salts

- 1/4 teaspoon oil (Lavender and Mandarin)

- 3/4 teaspoon liquid (evenly spread out through sprays)

- 1 drop of purple/orange food coloring

2. Summer Winds

You know that feeling you get when it's summer and you have laundry drying out in the back, and all of a sudden this sharp wind passes by and you can practically smell summer in the air?

For this recipe you are going to need -

- 2 tablespoons baking soda

- 1/2 tablespoon cream of tartar

- 1 tablespoon of cornstarch

- 1 tablespoon Epsom salts

- 1/4 teaspoon oil (Grapefruit, Lemon and Spearmint)

- 3/4 teaspoon liquid (evenly spread out through sprays)

- 1 drop of green food coloring

3. Autumn in Ney York

If you are a Manhattan-ite you know exactly how good a good soak can feel right in the middle of a New York Autumn, all those holiday's and people going back home to their families, it can be pretty amazing!

For this recipe you are going to need -

- 2 tablespoons baking soda

- 1/2 tablespoon cream of tartar

- 1 tablespoon of cornstarch

- 1 tablespoon Epsom salts

- 1/4 teaspoon oil (Cinnamon, Nutmeg, Clove Bud and Juniper Berry)

- 3/4 teaspoon liquid (evenly spread out through sprays)

- 1 drop of red/orange food coloring

4. Winter Wonderland

Is there anything more captivating than the sight of a beautiful white winter? Well maybe the winter wonderland bath bombs!

For this recipe you are going to need -

- 2 tablespoons baking soda

- 1/2 tablespoon cream of tartar

- 1 tablespoon of cornstarch

- 1 tablespoon Epsom salts

- 1/4 teaspoon oil (Ginger, Orange and Nutmeg)

- 3/4 teaspoon liquid (evenly spread out through sprays)

5. Rainy Day Special

Ever just had a long day and then walked out of work only to get soaked in the pouring rain? Sounds pretty awful but that doesn't mean it's the end of the world the rainy day special is to help chase away all your gloom!

For this recipe you are going to need -

- 2 tablespoons baking soda

- 1/2 tablespoon cream of tartar

- 1 tablespoon of cornstarch

- 1 tablespoon Epsom salts

- 1/4 teaspoon oil (Bergamot, Mint and Mandarin)

- 3/4 teaspoon liquid (evenly spread out through sprays)

Citric Acid Bases

All of the recipes that follow make exactly one bath bomb each, so feel free to alternate the recipe as needed!

6. The Bad Boss-day Bomb

For this recipe you are going to need -

- 2 tablespoons baking soda

- 1 tablespoon citric acid

- 1 tablespoon of cornstarch

- 1 tablespoon Epsom salts

- 1/4 teaspoon oil (Jasmine, Sweet Orange and Roman Chamomile)

- 3/4 teaspoon liquid (evenly spread out through sprays)

- 1 drop of purple food coloring

7. Down with the Blues

For this recipe you are going to need -

- 2 tablespoons baking soda

- 1 tablespoon citric acid

- 1 tablespoon of cornstarch

- 1 tablespoon Epsom salts

- 1/4 teaspoon oil (Clary Sage, Helichrysum and Patchouli)

- 3/4 teaspoon liquid (evenly spread out through sprays)

- 1 drop of blue food coloring

8. Anywhere but Here

For this recipe you are going to need -

- 2 tablespoons baking soda

- 1 tablespoon citric acid

- 1 tablespoon of cornstarch

- 1 tablespoon Epsom salts

- 1/4 teaspoon oil (Cypress, Palo Santo and Frankincense)

- 3/4 teaspoon liquid (evenly spread out through sprays)

- 1 drop of red/blue food coloring

9. Lost without You

For this recipe you are going to need -

- 2 tablespoons baking soda

- 1 tablespoon citric acid

- 1 tablespoon of cornstarch

- 1 tablespoon Epsom salts

- 1/4 teaspoon oil (Rose and Vetiver)

- 3/4 teaspoon liquid (evenly spread out through sprays)

- a smattering of dried rose petals

10. Happy Days

For this recipe you are going to need -

- 2 tablespoons baking soda

- 1 tablespoon citric acid

- 1 tablespoon of cornstarch

- 1 tablespoon Epsom salts

- 1/4 teaspoon oil (Geranium and Lemon)

- 3/4 teaspoon liquid (evenly spread out through sprays)

- 1 drop of yellow food coloring

11. *Forever Yours*

For this recipe you are going to need -

- 2 tablespoons baking soda

- 1 tablespoon citric acid

- 1 tablespoon of cornstarch

- 1 tablespoon Epsom salts

- 1/4 teaspoon oil (Hyssop and Rose)

- 3/4 teaspoon liquid (evenly spread out through sprays)

- 1 drop of orange and red food coloring

12. And ode to St. Valentine

For this recipe you are going to need -

- 2 tablespoons baking soda

- 1 tablespoon citric acid

- 1 tablespoon of cornstarch

- 1 tablespoon Epsom salts

- 1/4 teaspoon oil (Rose, Sandalwood, Mandarin and Jasmine)

- 3/4 teaspoon liquid (evenly spread out through sprays)

- a smattering of dried rose petals

13. Pride Parade

For this recipe you are going to need -

- 2 tablespoons baking soda

- 1 tablespoon citric acid

- 1 tablespoon of cornstarch

- 1 tablespoon Epsom salts

- 1/4 teaspoon oil (Bay Laurel, Grapefruit and Sweet Orange)

- 3/4 teaspoon liquid (evenly spread out through sprays)

- 1 drop of purple food coloring

14. Down By the Beach

For this recipe you are going to need -

- 2 tablespoons baking soda

- 1 tablespoon citric acid

- 1 tablespoon of cornstarch

- 1 tablespoon Epsom salts

- 1/4 teaspoon oil (Petitgrain, Sweet Orange, and Ylang Ylang)

- 3/4 teaspoon liquid (evenly spread out through sprays)

- 1 drop of yellow food coloring

15. The Last Bath

For this recipe you are going to need -

- 2 tablespoons baking soda

- 1 tablespoon citric acid

- 1 tablespoon of cornstarch

- 1 tablespoon Epsom salts

- 1/4 teaspoon oil (Eucalyptus and Lemon)

- 3/4 teaspoon liquid (evenly spread out through sprays)

- 1 drop of red/blue food coloring

16. The Taj Mahal

For this recipe you are going to need -

- 2 tablespoons baking soda

- 1/2 tablespoon cream of tartar

- 1 tablespoon of cornstarch

- 1 tablespoon Epsom salts

- 1/4 teaspoon oil (Jasmine and Sandalwood)

- 3/4 teaspoon liquid (evenly spread out through sprays)

17. Because You're Beautiful

For this recipe you are going to need -

- 2 tablespoons baking soda

- 1/2 tablespoon cream of tartar

- 1 tablespoon of cornstarch

- 1 tablespoon Epsom salts

- 1/4 teaspoon oil (Cedar wood and Spearmint)

- 3/4 teaspoon liquid (evenly spread out through sprays)

- 1 drop of green food coloring

18. Breakfast at Tiffany's

For this recipe you are going to need -

- 2 tablespoons baking soda

- 1/2 tablespoon cream of tartar

- 1 tablespoon of cornstarch

- 1 tablespoon Epsom salts

- 1/4 teaspoon oil (Cinnamon, Lime and Lavender)

- 3/4 teaspoon liquid (evenly spread out through sprays)

- 1 drop of green and blue food coloring

19. All Spice

For this recipe you are going to need -

- 2 tablespoons baking soda

- 1/2 tablespoon cream of tartar

- 1 tablespoon of cornstarch

- 1 tablespoon Epsom salts

- 1/4 teaspoon oil (Cinnamon, Sage, Neroli and Nutmeg)

- 3/4 teaspoon liquid (evenly spread out through sprays)

20. Sugary Sweet!

For this recipe you are going to need -

- 2 tablespoons baking soda

- 1/2 tablespoon cream of tartar

- 1 tablespoon of cornstarch

- 1 tablespoon Epsom salts

- 1/4 teaspoon oil (Vanilla, Sweet Orange and Cinnamon)

- 3/4 teaspoon liquid (evenly spread out through sprays)

21. Cabin in the Woods

For this recipe you are going to need -

- 2 tablespoons baking soda

- 1 tablespoon citric acid

- 1 tablespoon of cornstarch

- 1 tablespoon Epsom salts

- 1/4 teaspoon oil (Spruce, Fir Needle and Juniper)

- 3/4 teaspoon liquid (evenly spread out through sprays)

- 1 drop of green food coloring

22. Summer Secrets

For this recipe you are going to need -

- 2 tablespoons baking soda

- 1 tablespoon citric acid

- 1 tablespoon of cornstarch

- 1 tablespoon Epsom salts

- 1/4 teaspoon oil (Jojoba, Rose, Beeswax and Lemongrass)

- 3/4 teaspoon liquid (evenly spread out through sprays)

- 1 drop of green food coloring

23. Shiver me Timber

For this recipe you are going to need -

- 2 tablespoons baking soda

- 1 tablespoon citric acid

- 1 tablespoon of cornstarch

- 1 tablespoon Epsom salts

- 1/4 teaspoon oil (Cypress, Peppermint, and Cedar wood)

- 3/4 teaspoon liquid (evenly spread out through sprays)

24. Soul Food

For this recipe you are going to need -

- 2 tablespoons baking soda

- 1 tablespoon citric acid

- 1 tablespoon of cornstarch

- 1 tablespoon Epsom salts

- 1/4 teaspoon oil (Chocolate, Vanilla and Cinnamon)

- 3/4 teaspoon liquid (evenly spread out through sprays)

- a smattering of dried rose petals

25. Mistletoe

For this recipe you are going to need -

- 2 tablespoons baking soda

- 1 tablespoon citric acid

- 1 tablespoon of cornstarch

- 1 tablespoon Epsom salts

- 1/4 teaspoon oil (Frankincense and Myrrh)

- 3/4 teaspoon liquid (evenly spread out through sprays)

- 1 drop of red food coloring

And there you go, thirty different recipes each it's own journey, and thankfully one you can enjoy from the comfort of your home!

Conclusion

I hope this book was able to help you effectively learn not only how to make your own homemade bath bombs in theory but also that all those little, mixing, moldings and storing techniques have allowed you to test out all those various bath bomb recipes you have been earing so much about

Now that you've done your reading the next step is to put it all into action and find out for yourself how many amazing bath bomb recipes you can actually replicate!

Thank you and good luck!

Did you like this book bundle?

If you liked this bundle (or if you didn't), I'd love to hear your feedback and if it helped you. I welcome all feedback and use it to make my books better, so please leave a review for the book on Amazon if you have 30 seconds:
https://www.amazon.com/Homemade-Beauty-Products-Beginners-Luxurious-ebook/dp/B00UHY8LRI

Questions? Concerns? Please email us at epicpublishingbooks[at]gmail.com.